DEADLY KARATE BLOWS

DEADLY KARATE BLOWS

The Medical Implications

By
Brian Adams

DISCLAIMER

Please note that the publisher of this instructional book is NOT RESPONSIBLE in any manner whatsoever for any injury which may occur by reading and/or following the instructions herein.

It is essential that before following any of the activities, physical or otherwise, herein described, the reader or readers should first consult his or her physician for advice on whether or not the reader or readers should embark on the physical activity described herein. Since the physical activities described herein may be too sophisticated in nature, it is *essential that a physician be consulted.*

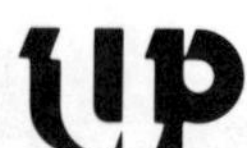

UNIQUE PUBLICATIONS
4201 VANOWEN PLACE, BURBANK, CA 91505

ISBN: 0-86568-077-9
Library of Congress Catalog Card Number: 86-50088

Published 1985. Printed in United States of America.

Designed by: Danilo J. Silverio

Dedication

This work was originally used as a thesis (part of the requirement) for black belt promotion in the International Kenpo Karate Association and was personally encouraged by Ed Parker, the president of the I.K.K.A. This book is dedicated to those who want to enjoy the art and science of karate, both physically and academically, for one without the other is only half an art.

Foreword

The art of karate as practiced today can be traced to ancient China. A pilgrim Buddhist monk is said to have taught an embryonic form of karate to his Chinese students in a Buddhist monastery in China. In 1600, the art as developed by this monk and his disciples was exported to Okinawa by Okinawan students of the Chinese art. The Okinawans took a keen interest in the art and combined it with a native form of hand to hand fighting to produce Okinawa-te. It was not until 1920 that karate was exported to Japan by an Okinawan school administrator and master of the art. Since that memorable event the Japanese style of the art has evolved to the point where it includes many systems.

Meanwhile, further evolution of the art was taking place in China, Okinawa, Korea, and Hawaii. More recently, the United States has become a "melting pot" of all the basic systems and a microcosm of the disputes concerned with discrepancies between theoretical and philosophical orientation and training procedures. One of the most pressing disputes involves the question of scored points during competition. Since there is little actual contact during karate competition, the effect cannot be directly observed. Anatomical points accepted as vital by one school of thought or system may not be recognized by another system. This type of controversy tends to prohibit competition between the groups and slow evolution of the art by limiting the scope of experience of tournament participants. Physical and anatomical theories generated years ago are tending to prevent open competition.

Unsupportable theory is indeed empty. Knowledge of anatomical fact seems to bear directly on the current controversy. What are the possible effects of a particular karate blow? What tissues and/or organs are involved? Twentieth-century medical and anatomical knowledge can answer these questions; but there is no published literature available, understandable to the non-professional, which applies even indirectly to karate. It is improbable that this vacuum of knowledge can be sustained without further damage to the art and its competitive aspects. The novice as well as the karate expert certainly would benefit by a more direct exposure to empirical anatomical facts researched from the karateist's perspective.

I have read a manuscript entitled *Deadly Karate Blows: The Medical Implications* written by Mr. Brian Adams, a black belt instructor. I feel that this manuscript represents a complete, well-illustrated, well-organized, sophisticated analysis of the medical aspects of basic karate blows and scientifically validated targets. I feel that distribution of Mr. Adams' work will satisfy most if not all of the needs on which I have commented above.

Sincerely,
ROBERT CHRISTOPHER TOWN,
Karate Instructor, Biology Teacher,
San Diego Military Academy,
San Diego, California

Preface

Although karate is an ancient art, it has only recently enjoyed a renaissance in the world at large, and in the United States in particular. Much has been written about the various *methods* of karate and the techniques involved. Little has been written on the *effects* of the many and varied karate blows. *Deadly Karate Blows: The Medical Implications* attempts to fill this gap.

Brian Adams has endeavored in this book to standardize the techniques of karate as to the bodily harm that may be inflicted by a particular blow. He accurately demonstrates the blow and then in great detail lists the likely injuries that would result from such an encounter.

The main interest of this work is the examination of the medical implications of a karate blow and not the strict execution of the technique involved. Considering this, two or three photographs were found to be adequate for demonstrating each technique. In addition, the individual Karate practitioner is certain to have his own preferred methods and theories of technique execution which we respect and do not wish to challenge.

Medical information for this work was accumulated through many years of direct study in the field and of course was substantiated and compounded thanks to the services of many technical advisors: physicians in general practice, physiologists, anaesthetists, surgeons, chiropractors, physiological psychologists, osteopaths and anatomists.

The main interest of this work is the examination of the medical implications of a karate blow and not the strict technique involved. Therefore only two or three photographs are used to demonstrate each technique discussed, but there are many accompanying anatomical and explanatory diagrams and drawings.

The blows used in this book are those familiar to most schools of karate. These blows include killing, paralyzing, and partially disabling blows in varying degrees of severity. Obviously this book will serve to familiarize students of karate with the intended purpose and result of the many maneuvers employed. The why and wherefore of the actions and their importance is made clear as they relate to the impact upon the human body. Furthermore, a sense of responsibility will be developed in the student as he comes to realize the possibility of inflicting serious injury upon others.

Probably the most important contribution of all will be to standardize the judging of karate matches. Since there is little actual contact during karate competition, effect cannot be directly observed. Anatomical points accepted as vital by one school or system may not be recognized by another system. At present there is on the market no standard medical or anatomical literature, understandable to the non-professional which even indirectly applies to karate.

A bibliography is included as an incentive for the reader's further investigation. It includes the main volumes used in the research and initial verification of medical information used here.

Nozawa Trading, Inc., of Los Angeles, California, donated the use of the reaction timing device which we used to measure the *total* reflex action time for each technique. The machine is calibrated in tenths of a second. We found that an intermediate student of the Brown Belt (SANKYU) category consistently completed each technique in less than nine-tenths of one second. (This figure includes the time used to execute any block, parry, or grab called for in the technique.)

A top view is used in some sections because sometimes a photo taken from the side will not show the exact angles of body torque, etc., applied in the technique, which is a very important factor when determining the exact angle struck on the human anatomy.

An oversimplification of anatomical drawings is used in many of the sections to keep from distracting the reader from the main point of interest.

Deadly Karate Blows: The Medical Implications thus represents a complete, well-organized, sophisticated analysis of the medical aspects of basic karate blows which will satisfy the needs of the professional enthusiast, as well as the spectator who only wishes to enjoy a rapidly growing sport.

About the Author

Brian Adams has been a martial art instructor, with his own self-defense school in San Diego, California, for nearly 25 years. He began his career in the karate world at the age of eighteen. At the time of his introduction to karate, he was majoring in psychology at Pasadena City College, California. To better understand the philosophies of oriental culture, he decided to begin his study with the deep intricacies of specific oriental societies; that basis stemming from one of the oldest practices of the Far East—karate (the oriental method of self-defense). As his studies progressed in the art, he began to realize the great physical and psychological values in karate training. Realizing that the western world is so full of everyday tensions and anxieties and because his life career would be dealing with people, he decided to help people relieve mental pressures by giving them a socially accepted way to "let off steam," and to throw a new light on self-realization and the life process (new to the western way of life, that is).

Recognized as an expert in the field of martial injuries, he has taught his programs at several universities and to the staff of California State hospitals. Mr. Adams has also served as an "Expert Witness" in criminal trials and Grand Jury hearings that dealt with martial art type assaults and injuries.

In 1984, Brian closed the doors of his school and now spends the majority of his time pursuing martial art research and development. His latest contribution is a sophisticated line of martial art training gear and devices.

The techniques in this book are demonstrated by two expert, experienced martial art teachers: Gilbert Martinez and Randy Williams. The photographer was Ed Ikuta.

Table of Contents

Introduction

With the introduction and acceptance of karate and all its related arts throughout the world, have come many legends, a great many of them dealing with the physiological possibilities of various type blows on the human anatomy. These legends from the past are very intriguing, but unscientific. In this modern age there are still many unanswered questions regarding the potential of a well-focused karate blow on its target. My goal is to try and stimulate a greater interest in the scientific aspect of the art of karate, with emphasis on the medical effects of karate blows.

Naturally, I have included blows familiar to most schools of karate. These blows include killing, paralyzing and partially disabling blows in varying degrees of severity. One must remember that whenever the human element is involved, there is no such thing as absolute perfection. This is why in many of the sections it is indicated that there is more than one possible result, because the blow may be slightly off target or because of other existing conditions which might be hindered by unforeseen circumstances.

It must be clearly understood that I have just barely scratched the surface of a subject that will continue to regain its status in the martial arts. I have dealt only with the common and uncomplicated phases of injury that can occur from a karate blow. I have purposely avoided the complications of different types of long-range infection, which may have been present before the injury took place or may (due to the weakened state of the individual or other preexisting forces) end in a later infection or disease. Incidentally, this may account for many of the existing mystical "Poison Hand" legends from China. Whether or not the Chinese knew through scientific means what could happen if certain targets were struck or knew through trial and error or by mystical practices no one can say for sure.

I sincerely hope that the knowledge in this book will not be misused by a minority of individuals preaching sensationalism in the arts but rather will be used by sincere instructors and students who are interested in furthering not only their physical ability but who are also devoted to going along with the tradition of the art by improving their knowledge of medicine through the understanding of anatomy, physics, trauma (injury) and first aid.

A section on the principles and legalities of first aid will be found at the end of the book. This supplementary section was added upon the sixth printing, due to the overwhelming number of requests by martial artists all over the world to know more about first aid principles.

1

Striking the Forehead

Against a club attack to the head, defender sidesteps to the outside and parries or redirects the momentum of the attacker's downward blow toward his thigh, bringing his head down and forward.

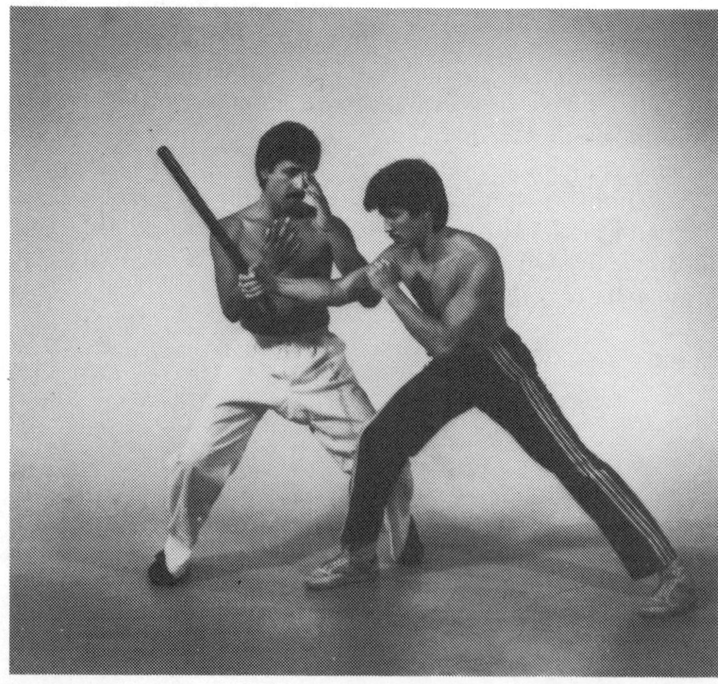

While holding his arm down, defender pivots into an elbow strike between the eyes. This technique was completed in 7/10 of one second.

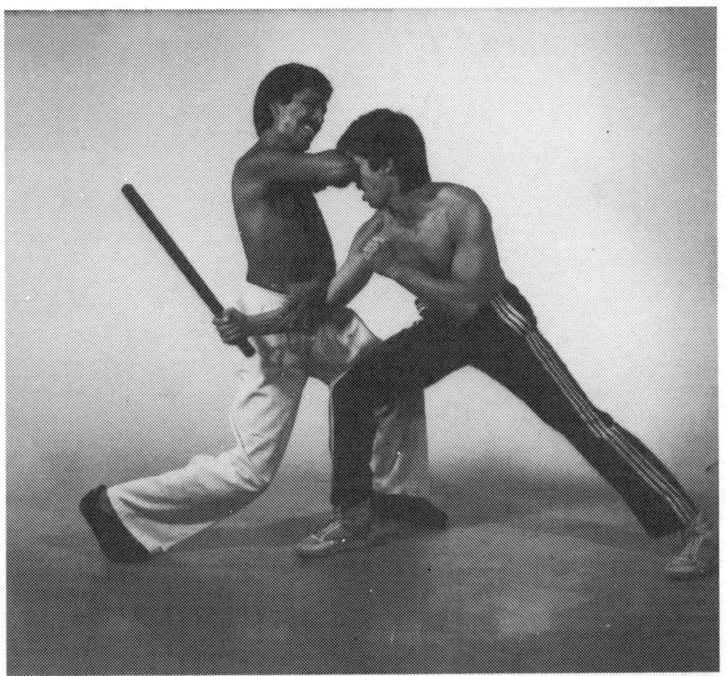

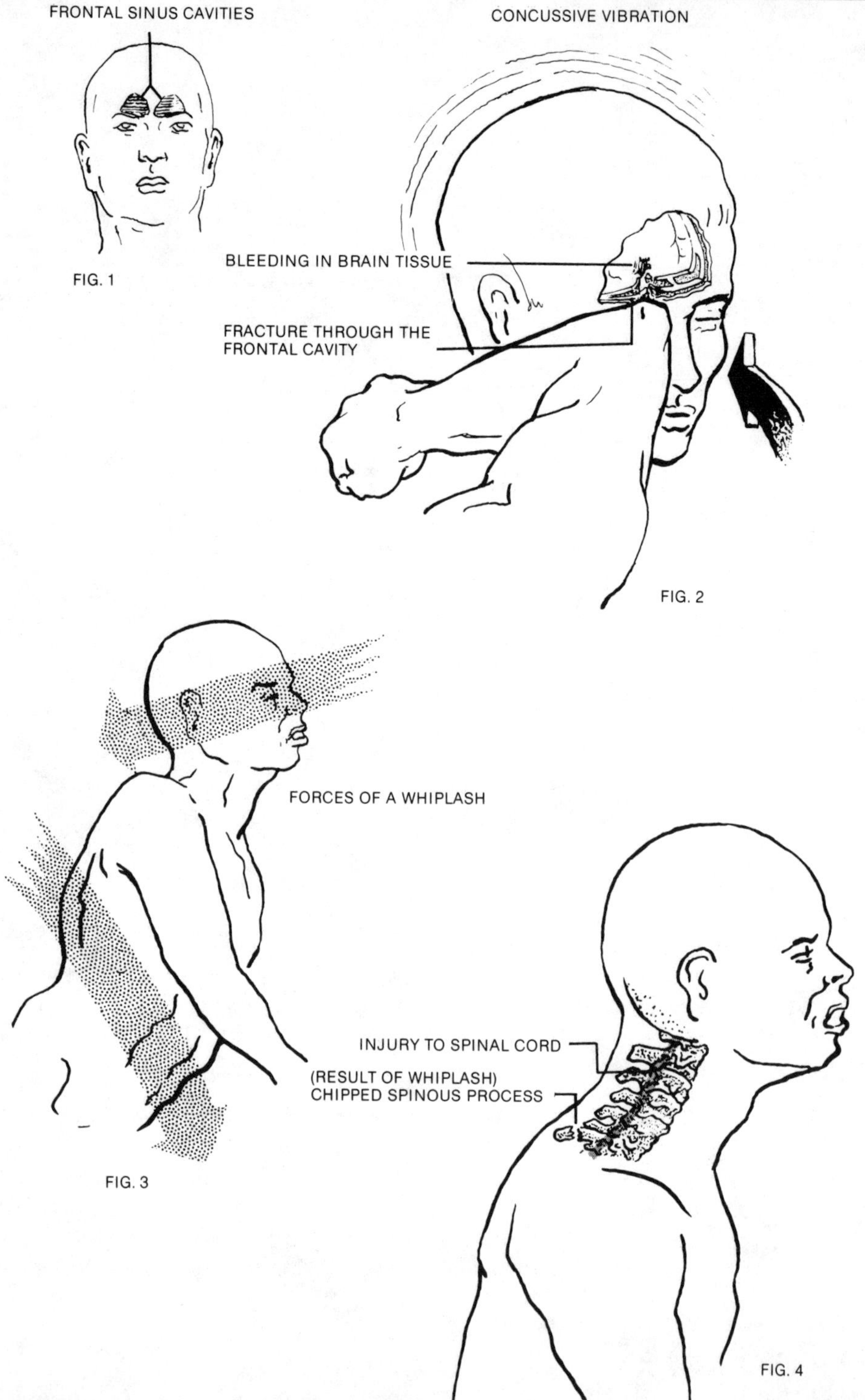

FIG. 1

FIG. 2

FIG. 3

FIG. 4

WEAPON: Elbow
TARGET: Middle of forehead

Medical Implications

I. TWO BLACK EYES would be the slightest possible effect due to the branching out pattern of the deep winding blood vessels in this region of the skull.

II. A LIGHT TO SEVERE CONCUSSION would occur assuming (*as we shall in all techniques presented in this work*) that all of the forces are moving well and in the right directions. In this case, the head would be moving down and forward into the oncoming elbow. This would increase the impact greatly and thereby increase the effectiveness of the blow by nearly one hundred per cent.

A "concussion" is the vibration (or shaking) of the brain within the brain case. The damage caused by such shaking can range from almost insignificant to certainly fatal results, depending upon the number of blood vessels ruptured and their positions relative to the brain itself.

Rupture of the vessels in the membrane (Dura) surrounding the brain or, more deeply, in the brain itself, will cause a brain hemorrhage and attendant blood clot. Such clots may cause immediate death or paralysis (as in a "stroke") or it may cause pressure to build up within the brain until "something gives." A really effective, well-focused elbow strike to the center of the forehead would be expected to run the gauntlet from unconsciousness and coma to death.

III. A SKULL FRACTURE OR A FRACTURE THROUGH THE FRONTAL SINUS (a small cavity above the eyebrow) would be one effect if the blow were struck slightly to one side or the other of the lower forehead. If the elbow strike were a follow-through type blow, it would cause the bone fragments of the first fracture to be driven through the back of the thin-boned wall of the sinus cavity and into the brain, causing bleeding there. There would also be profuse bleeding from the nostrils because of the tearing of mucous membrane linings in the sinus cavity. These results will cause immediate unconsciousness, coma, and most certainly death.

IV. A WHIPLASH INJURY would occur due to the quick change of head position. (First the head would lean forward and down and then it would be suddenly snapped straight back while the rest of the body was still moving in the opposite direction). With this action, one of the vertebral tips (spinous process) might be forced against a larger tip and be completely chipped off the vertebra, resulting in extreme pain and stiffness of the neck.

2

Striking the Ears

Against a two hand push, defender steps back and scoops downward and out, bringing opponent's torso down and forward.

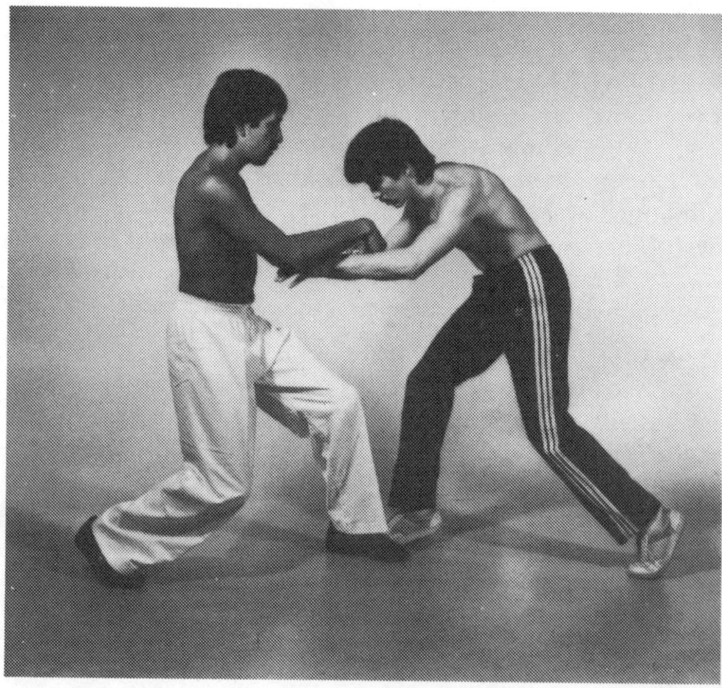

Defender carries the momentum of the scoop into the blow, directed to the ears with cupped hands. This technique was completed in 7/10 of one second.

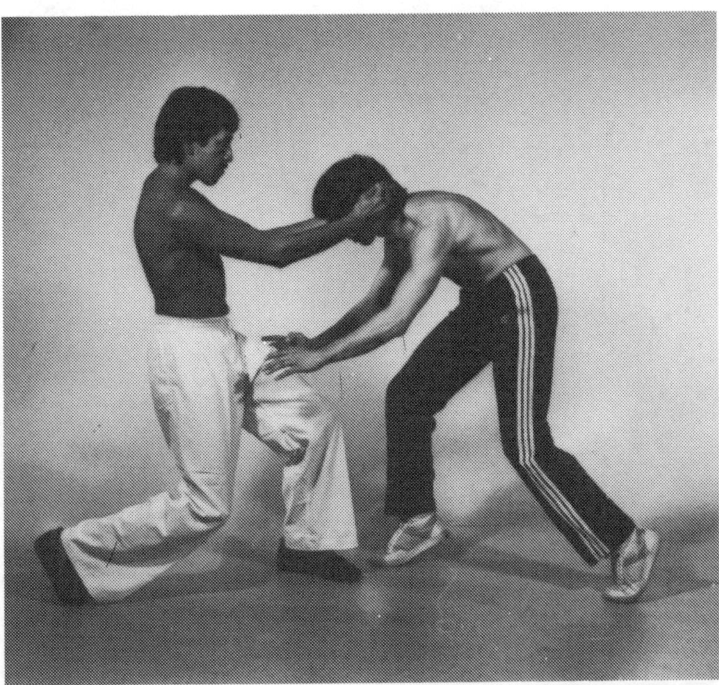

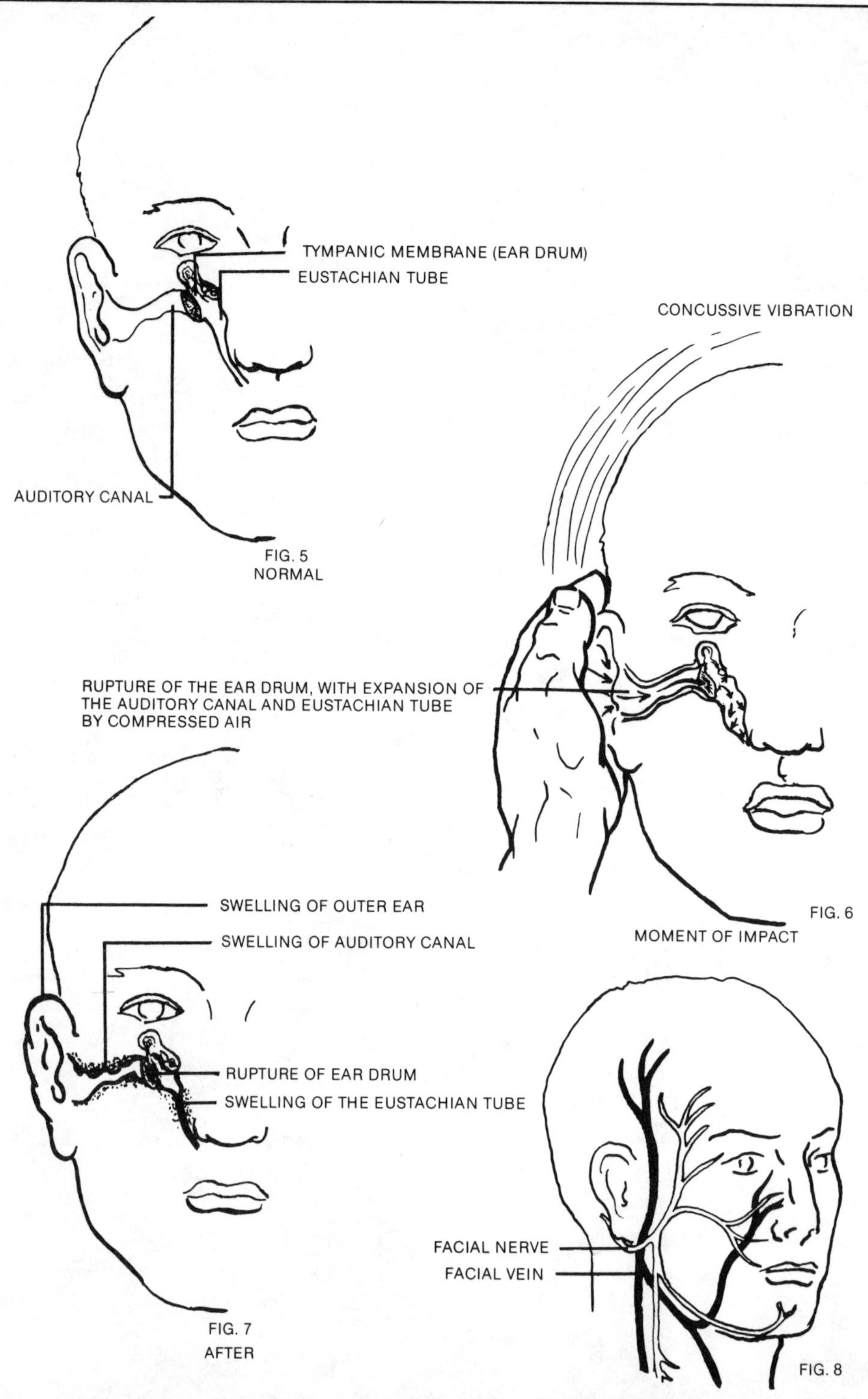

FIG. 5
NORMAL

FIG. 6
MOMENT OF IMPACT

FIG. 7
AFTER

FIG. 8

WEAPON: Cupped Palms
TARGET: Ears

Medical Implications

I. UNCONSCIOUSNESS OR A CONCUSSION will occur from any well-focused blow to the head. This is especially true when the head is not allowed to roll with the blow. The palms striking on both sides of the head simultaneously will act as a stabilizing device to the head and therefore doubles the percussive shock and pain. *Whenever there is the possibility of a concussion there is the possibility of death.*

II. RUPTURE OF THE TYMPANAC MEMBRANE (Eardrum) will result from the large volume of air being forced through the external auditory canal, through the thin-skinned membrane of the eardrum, and finally through the eustachian tube which opens into the back of the throat. The outside of the ear will be swollen because of the broken blood vessels and small capillaries there. Capillaries inside the auditory canal will be ruptured and swell because of the expanding volume of air that has rushed through the narrow passageway leading to the eardrum. Loss of hearing would be from partial to complete, depending upon the total degree of injury to the internal ear. The eustachian tube is much narrower than the auditory canal (the size of a pencil lead), and therefore will suffer greater expanding pressures as the air passes through it. The eustachian tube will undoubtedly swell completely shut. There will be an extreme amount of pain from the double palm strike to the ears. If the blows are not pulled, shock will be a prominent result.

III. POSSIBLE FRACTURE AND/OR DISLOCATION OF THE JAW HINGE (refer to Fig. 24) may occur if the blow is slightly lower.

IV. CONTUSION OF THE FACIAL NERVE AND VEIN, with possible paralysis of one side of the face, are experienced if the blow abrades them against the edge of the jawbone. This paralysis would probably be temporary unless a sharp section of the bone fracture punctured or severed the facial nerve. Likewise, if the vein was punctured there would be a small hematoma* (walnut-size lump) and eventually one side of the face would turn black and blue. (Fig. 8.)

* HEMATOMA: An organized area of blood spilled from a torn blood vessel.

3

Striking the Temple

Against a horizontal club strike to the head, defender steps in and executes a double block to opponent's arm.

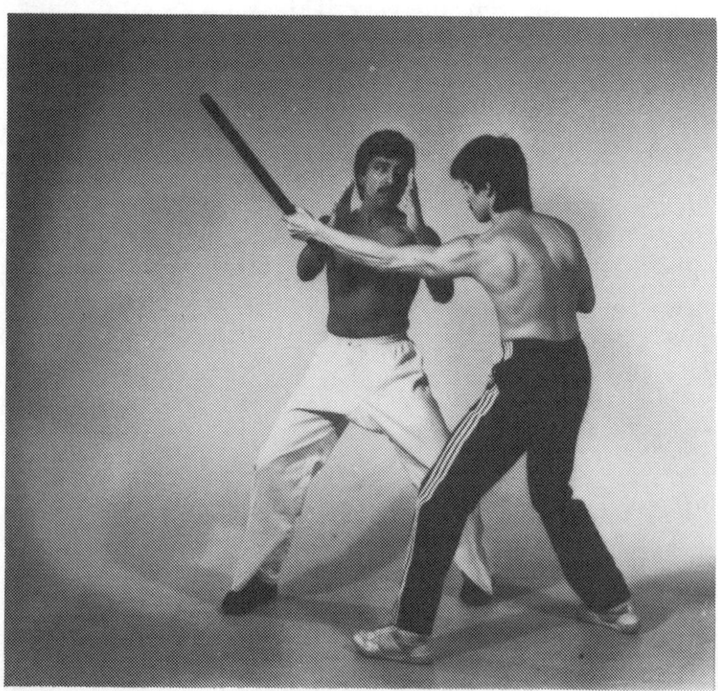

The right hand grabs the armed hand and pulls forward. Left hand executes a back knuckle to opponent's temple. This technique was completed in 8/10 of one second.

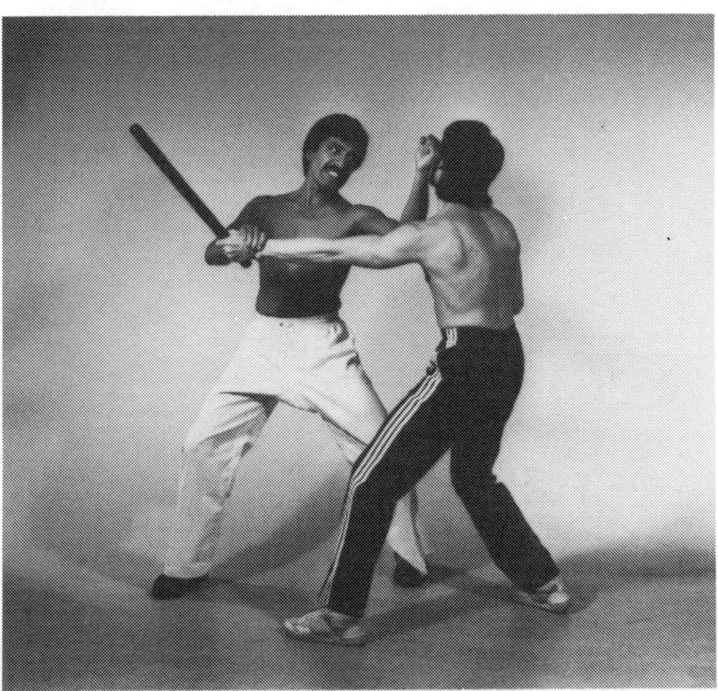

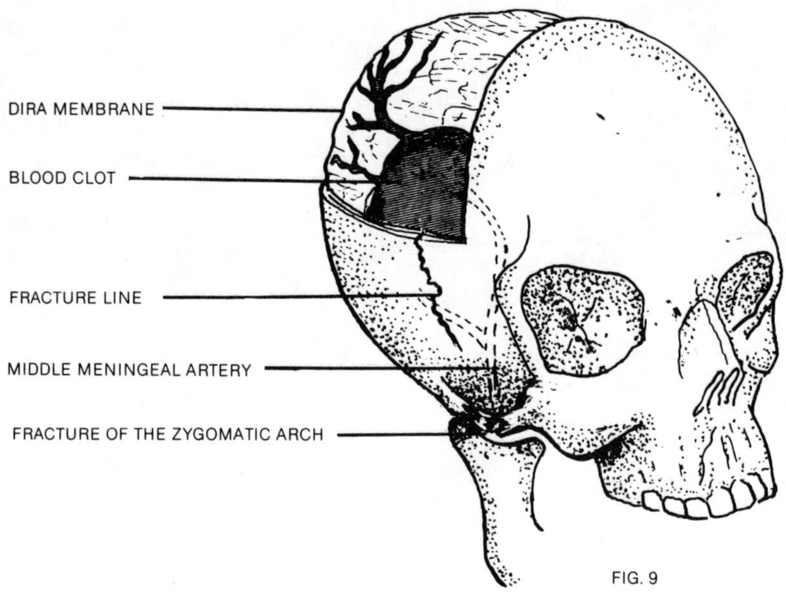

FIG. 9

FIG. 10 BLOW UP OF VEIN GROOVED INTO THE DURA MEMBRANE AND INSIDE THE SKULL

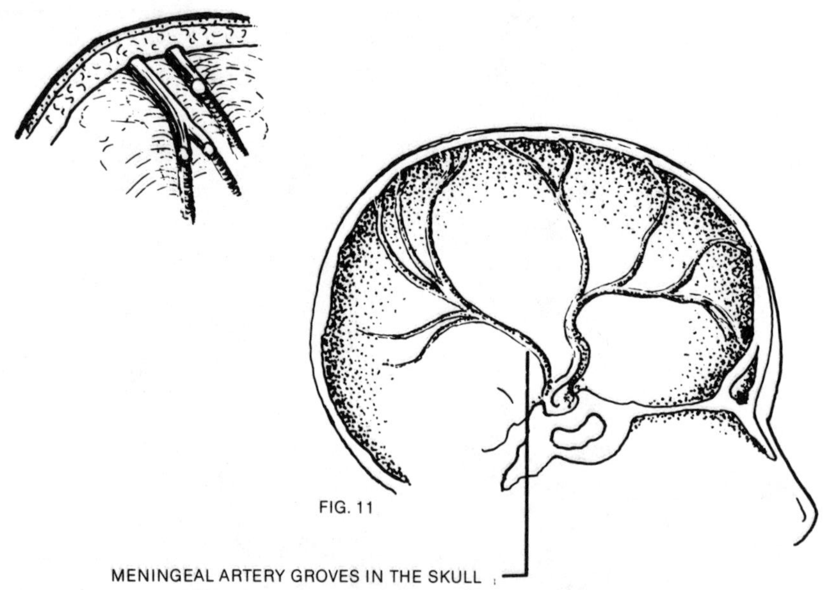

FIG. 11

WEAPON: Back-knuckle
TARGET: Temple

Medical Implications

I. A FRACTURE IN THE TEMPORAL REGION OF THE SKULL WITH MIDDLE MENINGEAL HEMORRHAGE (Meningeal Artery) commonly occur together; however, one may prevail without the other. The meningeal artery supplies the skull and dura (membrane that covers the brain) with blood. The artery follows its groove in the skull case (Fig. 10) and is easily pinched or severed if disruption of this groove occurs from a skull fracture.

II. HEADACHE, NAUSEA, VOMITING, COMA AND DEATH may ensue immediately or may be the delayed result, as long as two weeks later. If the artery were severed there would be immediate compression of the brain due to the massive hemorrhage there, indicated by a gradual deepening stupor. If diagnosis is not made soon, the patient will go into a coma and finally death will result. If the artery is only pinched with slow blood leakage, a small extradural hematoma* will produce delayed results, similar to a complete severence of the meningeal artery. Rupture of the meningeal artery may be prevailent without an accompanying skull fracture due to the severe jarring action displacing the vein from its groove. (Refer to Chapter 1)

III. RUPTURE OF THE TYMPANIC MEMBRANE (EARDRUM) may occur if the fracture line runs through the internal ear section of the skull. This will be evident from bleeding of the ear, nose, and mouth, and also from the vomiting of blood that has been swallowed and an obvious impairment of hearing.

IV. A FRACTURE OF THE ZYGOMATIC PROCESS will be the outcome if the blow is one inch lower than the temporal bone (temple). Opening and closing of the mouth will be noticeably painful. (Fig. 9.)

* Extradural hematoma: Blood clot between the skull casing and the dura.

4

Striking the Eye

Against a straight jab, defender steps back and parries opponent's arm to the outside.

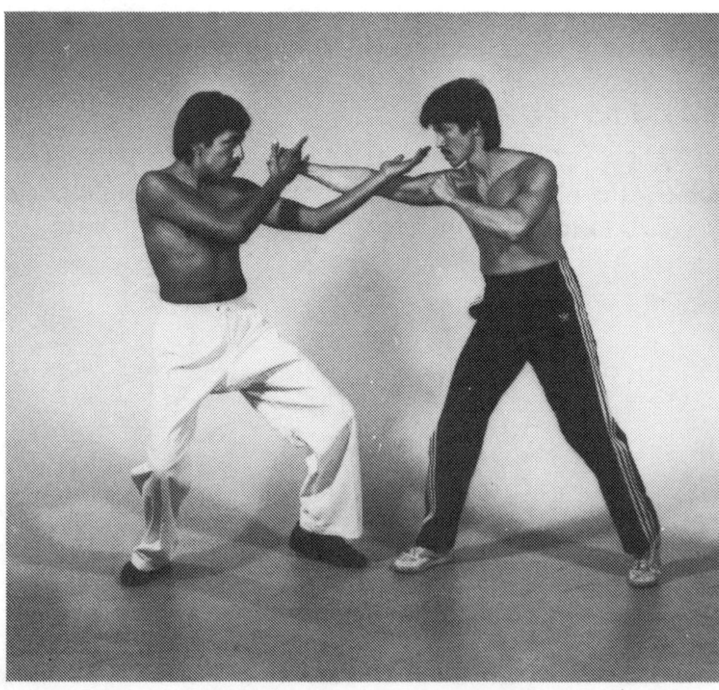

Defender immediately thrusts forward with fingers of left hand into opponent's eyes while right hand guards against the jab. This technique was completed in 5/10 of one second.

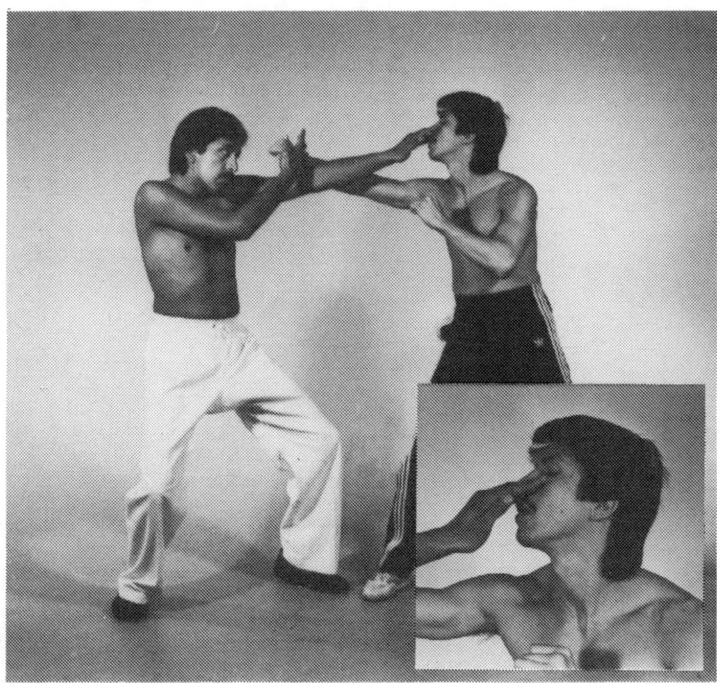

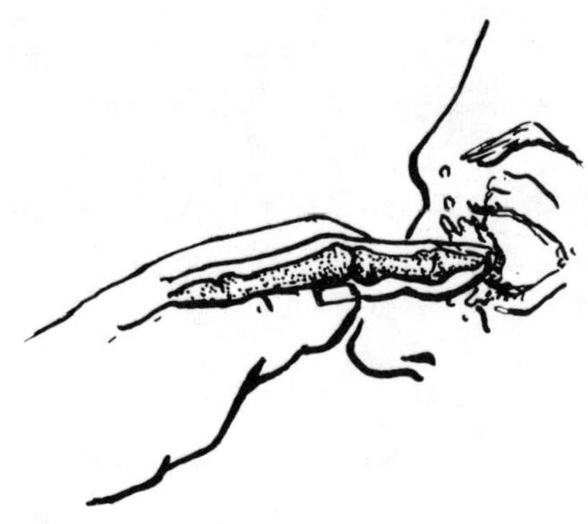
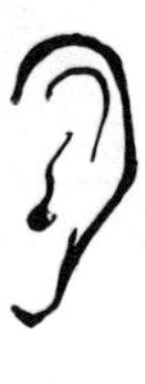

FIG. 12
COLLAPSED BULB OF EYE

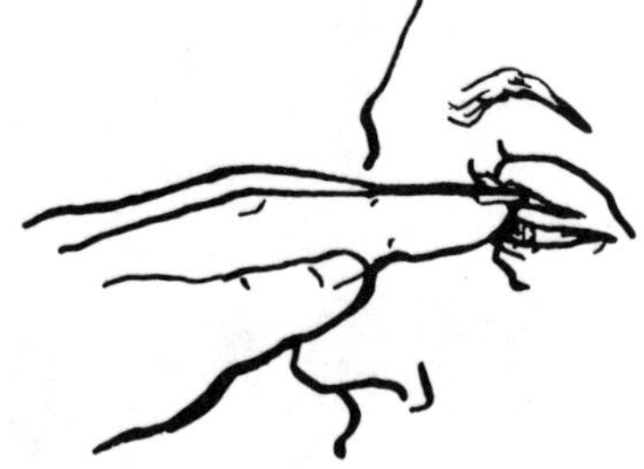
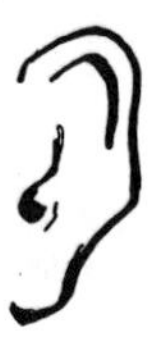

FIG. 13
LACERATED EYE LID

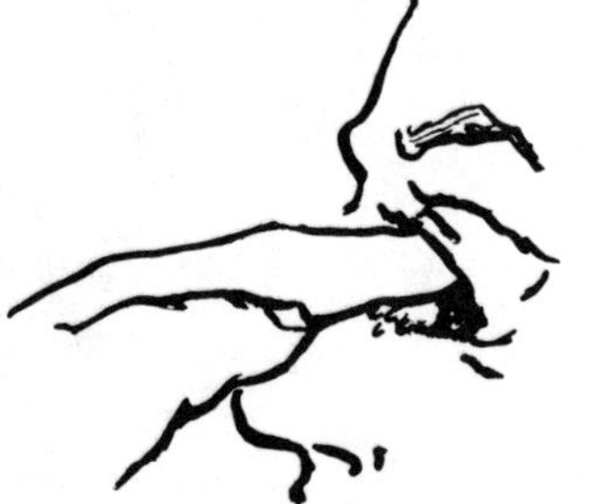
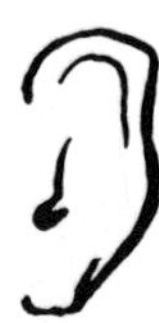

FIG.14
COLLAPSED BULB OF EYE

WEAPONS: Finger tips
TARGET: Eye

Medical Implications

I. The possible results are so many in this area, that we will concern ourselves with only the more obvious trauma.

RUPTURE OF THE EYE BULB WITH PROTRUSION OF THE WATERY AND GELATINOUS LIKE CONTENTS will result when the bulb is no longer able to withstand the direct pressure piercing it.

TEMPORARY TO PERMANENT BLINDNESS (Probably permanent) is the common result. Tremendous shocking pain will prevail in one or both eyes. An uncontrollable watering of the eyes will always be functional whenever a foreign object enters or touches the eye, which naturally produces temporary blurred vision in the uninjured eye.

II. A TORN EYELID (usually the top one, Fig. 13) is the effect of a sharp fingernail piercing an eyelid that has blinked at the last instant before the nail has struck.

Infection following trauma of this kind is the usual aftermath because of small debris (dirt, germs, hair, etc.) that enters the eye with the finger and nail. Sometimes infection can be a more serious complication than the blow itself.

5

Striking the Bridge of the Nose

Against a right cross, defender steps back and blocks the blow to the outside with the cocked left arm.

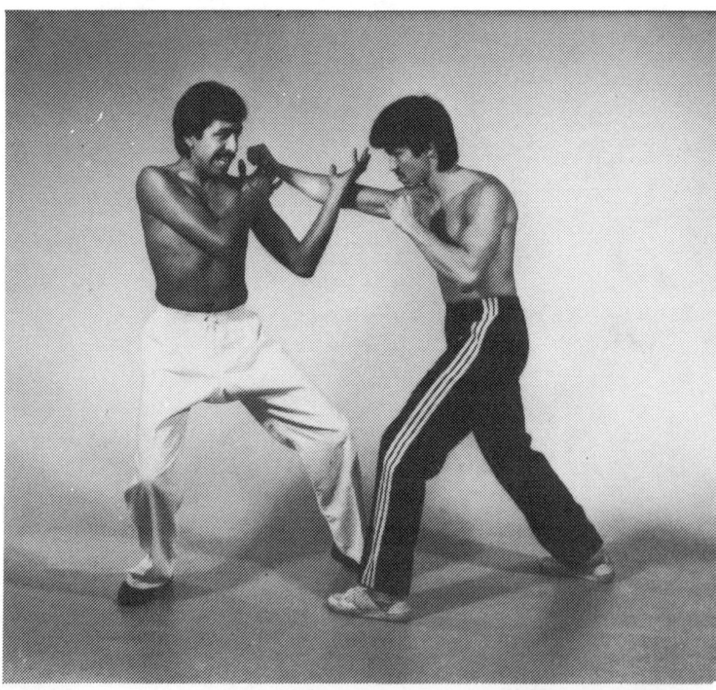

Moving forward for power, defender rakes the knuckles of left fist against opponent's nose. This technique was completed in 6/10 of one second.

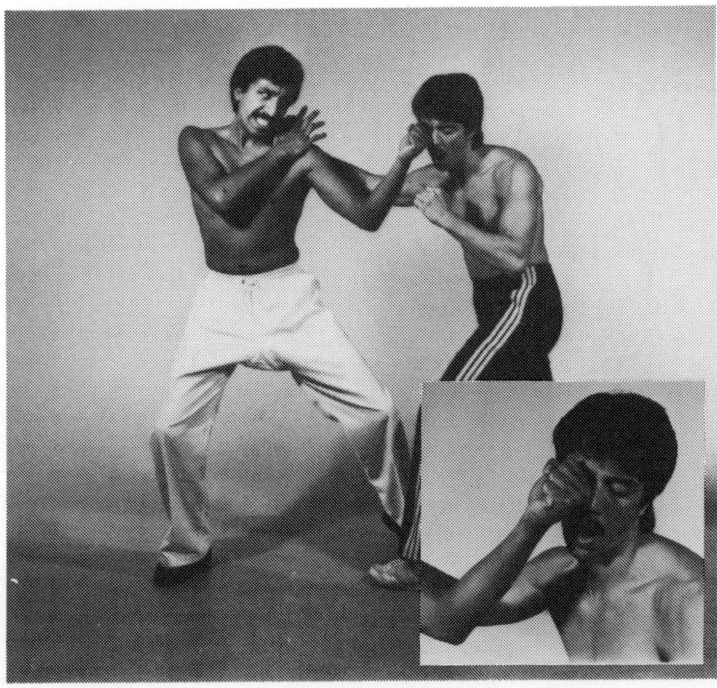

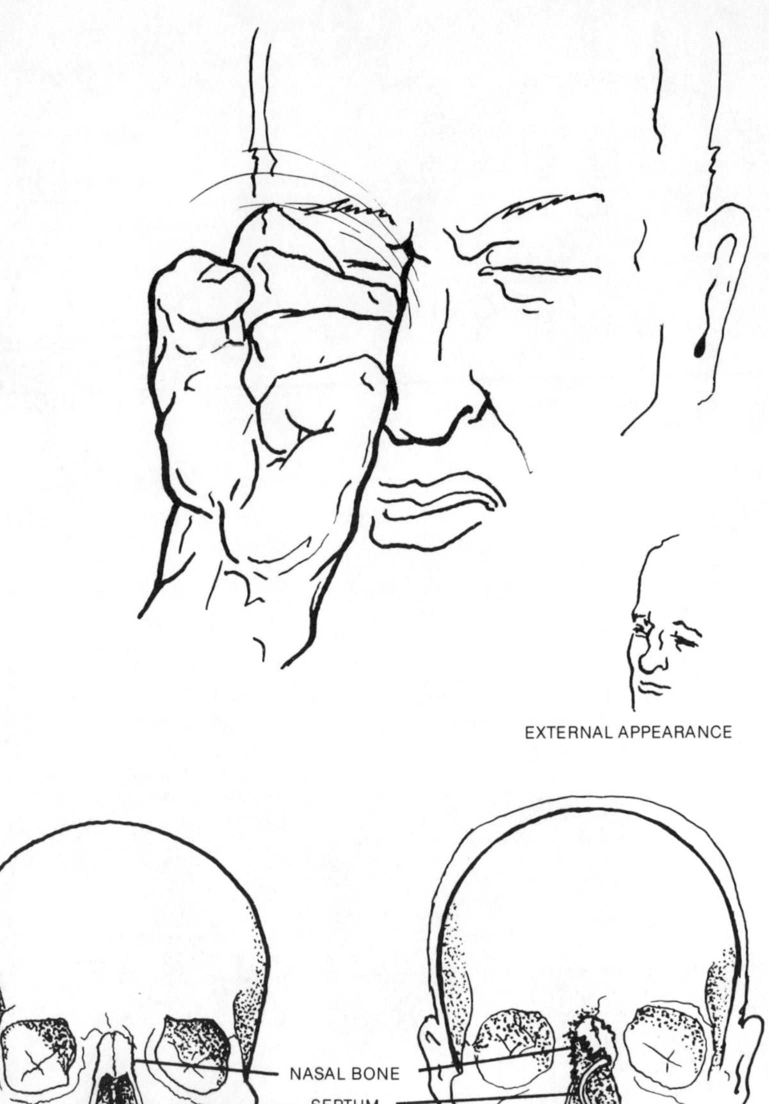

NORMAL

FIG. 15

FRACTURE AND DISLOCATION OF THE NASAL BONE AND SEPTUM (CARTILAGE THAT DIVIDES THE SIDES OF THE NOSTRILS)

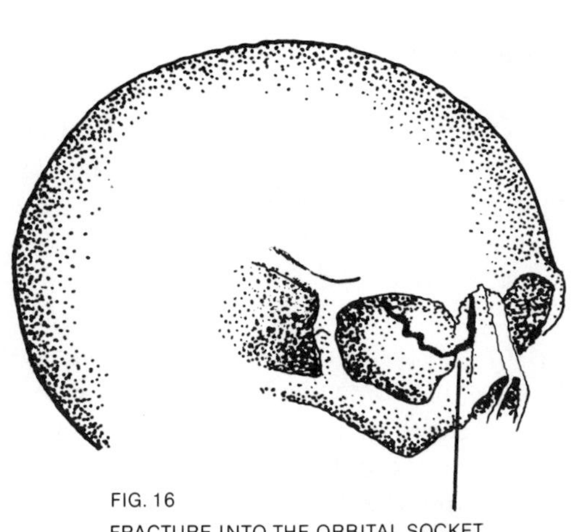

FIG. 16

FRACTURE INTO THE ORBITAL SOCKET

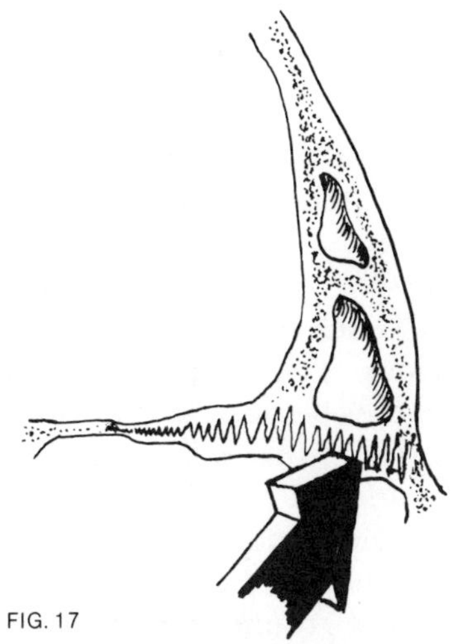

FIG. 17

OSOLATIONS FOLLOW PATH OF LEAST RESISTANCE AND BECOME CLOSER TOGETHER AS THE BONE NARROWS

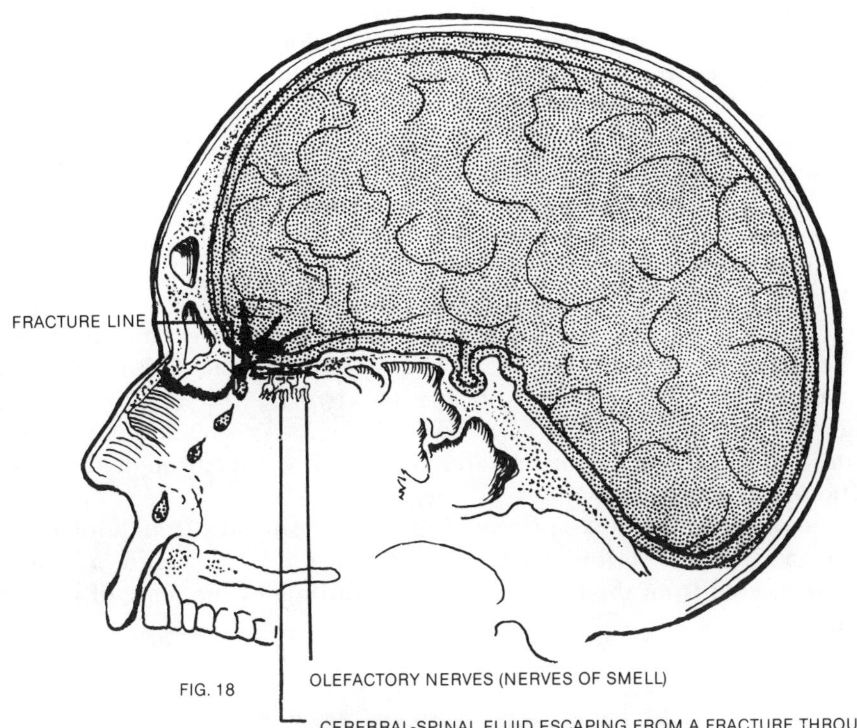

FIG. 18

WEAPONS: Back of all four knuckles
TARGET: Nasal bone

Medical Implications

I. A COMPOUND FRACTURE AND/OR DISLOCATION OF THE NASAL BONE AND SEPTUM (dividing partition of the nostrils) are a consequence of all four knuckles raking across the upper part of the nose. Needless to say, there will be massive hemorrhage because of the many blood vessels in this area. Shock and pain may render your opponent unconscious. Temporary blindness may be a result of the extreme watering of the eyes because of the stimulated pain receptors in the nasal region. We must realize that many times the blow may not be a death-dealing one, but the accidental consequences may end in death. In this case we are talking about unconsciousness which invariably occurs before the opponent hits the ground. The effect is a grave one because the head is relaxed when it strikes the ground and may end in a serious concussion or skull fracture if the surface is fairly solid. (Refer to Chapter 1.) Death may also ensue because of the huge amount of blood clogging the trachea (wind pipe) during unconsciousness.

II. FRACTURE INTO THE ORBITAL SOCKET (eye socket) with possible cerebral involvement may be a complication of the blow. If the fracture line has continued into the brain casing (cribriform plate of the ethmoid bone), a slight tear in the dura will release small amounts of cerebrospinal fluid. The fluid will travel through the sinuses and finally exit through the nostrils or be swallowed. Cerebrospinal fluid (clear fluid that circulates in the closed cavity of the brain and spinal cord) is sometimes mistaken for a normal secretion for quite some time, until severe headaches motivate the individual to seek medical advice.

When bone (or for that matter any part of the body) is struck, the force of the blow is transferred from the weapon to the target in the form of oscillating vibrations. In the case of bone the oscillations follow the path of least resitence. The oscillations are further apart in wide or thick bone and closer together in thin or narrow bone (Fig. 17). As oscillations narrow the vibration becomes more violent and causes a fracture through the weakest portion of bone.

The olefactory nerves (nerves of smell) are spread throughout the roof of the nasal section (cribiform plate of the ethmoid bone) and may become torn or severed from the fractured bone. A dulling of the sense of smell will occur.

6
Striking the Spot Under the Nose

Opponent has grabbed left wrist with right hand and prepares for attack with left hook.

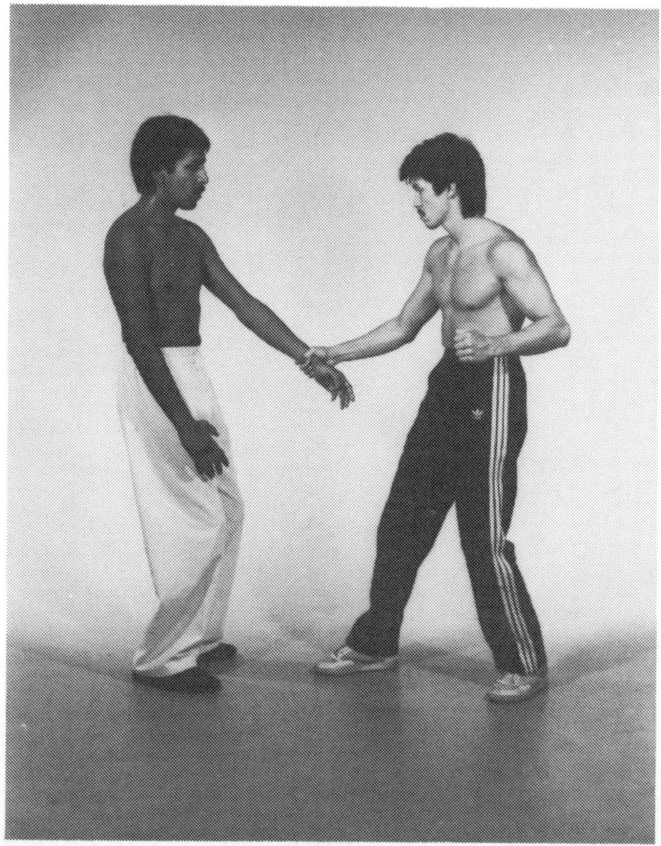

Defender steps in and simultaneously swings captured wrist across body, counter-grabbing opponent's wrist, and twisting hand free.

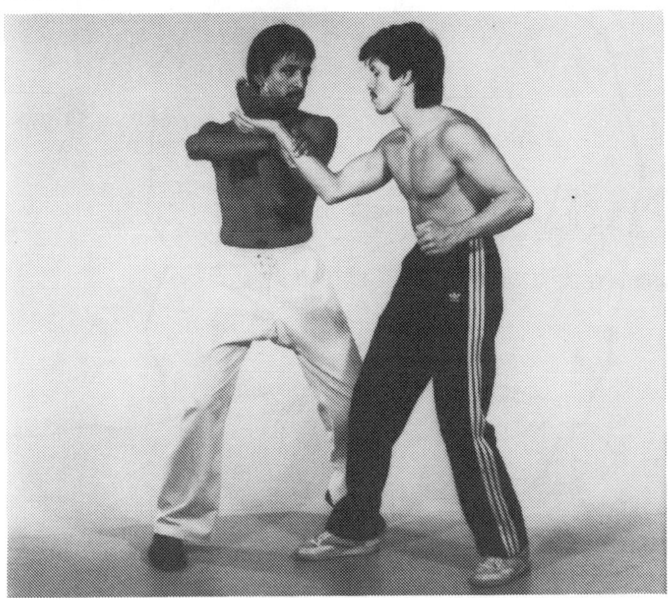

Defender pulls the attacker's arm while striking with a chop under attacker's nose. This technique was completed in 5/10 of one second.

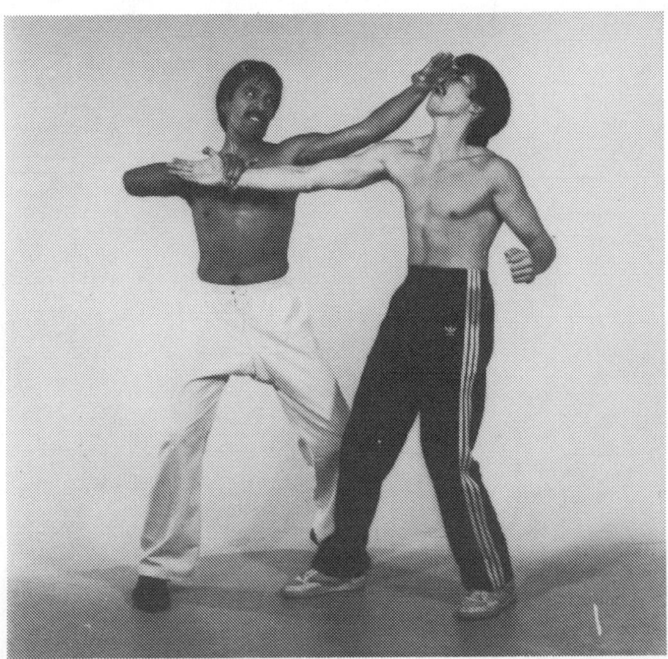

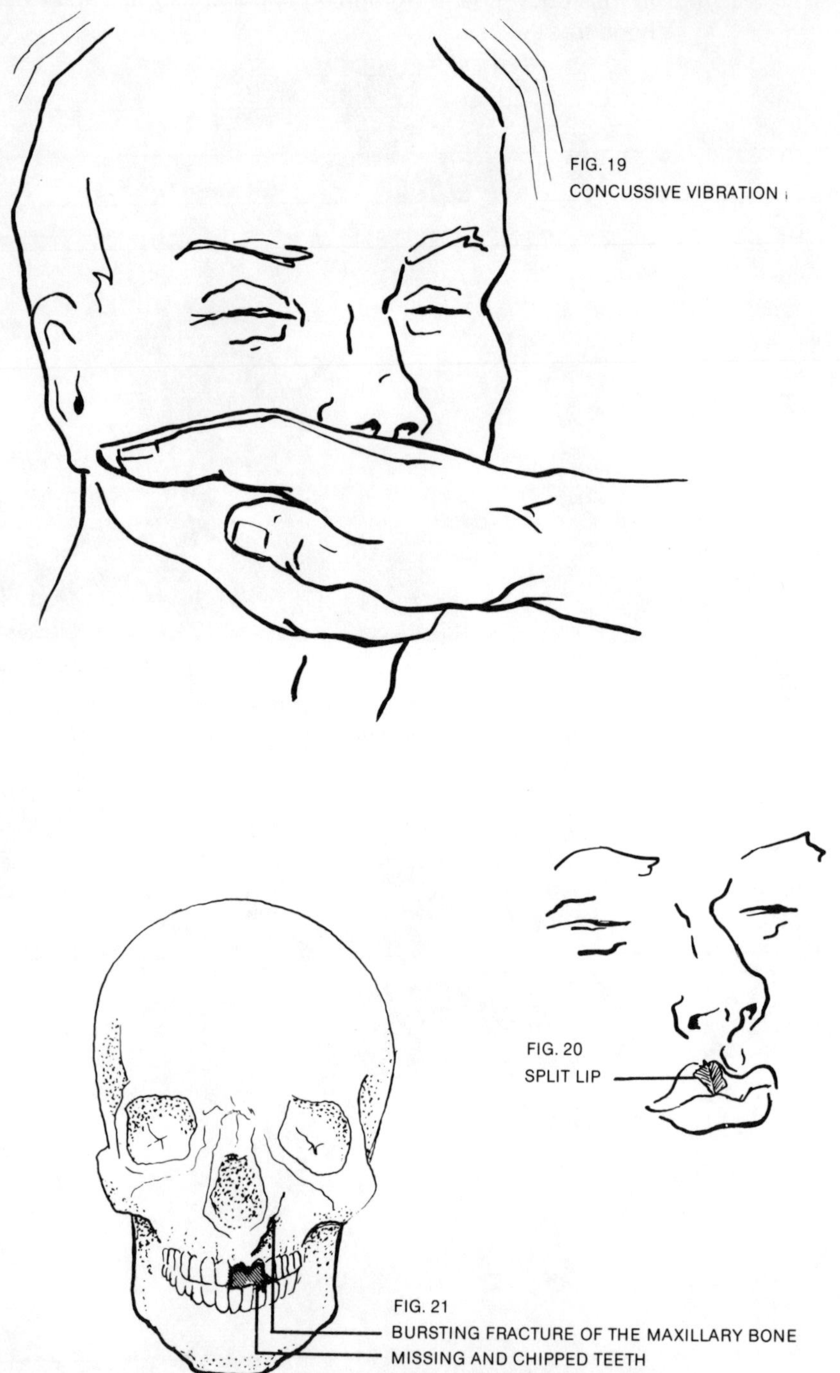

FIG. 19
CONCUSSIVE VIBRATION

FIG. 20
SPLIT LIP

FIG. 21

WEAPON: Chop (side of the hand)
TARGET: Region under the nose

Medical Implications

I. A SPLIT LIP, CHIPPED OR MISSING TEETH AND EYEWATERING PAIN are the minimal possible results. The eyewatering pain is due to the close proximity of the nerves to the surface of the skin.

II. A BURSTING FRACTURE OF THE MAXILLA (upper jaw) is the outcome because of the spherical nature of the skull. The skull will compress to its limit and then burst, producing a bursting fracture. The fracture site is usually on one side or the other, distal to the point of impact, but there may be a fracture at the impact site also. The simple task of eating may become a very painful one.

III. UNCONSCIOUSNESS AND/OR CONCUSSION frequently follow such a blow. (Refer to Chapter 1.) Unconsciousness may be a result of a concussion or more than likely may be caused by the fast exit of blood from the brain into the internal organs (due to shock).

IV. RESPIRATORY PARALYSIS AND DEATH may develop from broken or dislocated teeth and blood caught in or near the wind pipe (trachea) may cause a spasm of the vocal cords (Fig. 30) with closing off of the air supply.

7

Striking the Jaw

Against a reverse punch, defender steps back to his right as he parries the punch to the left.

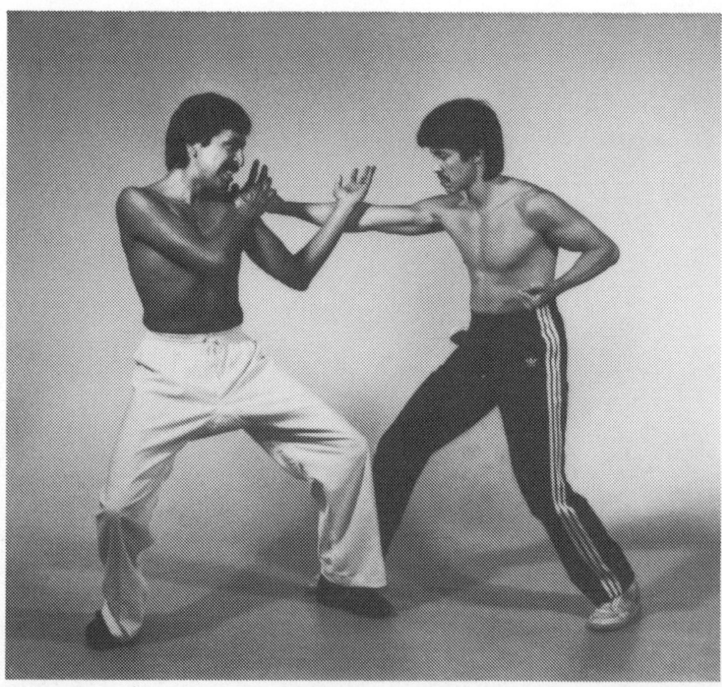

Defender steps in with simultaneous heel-of-the-palm and elbow strike to the jaw. This technique was completed in 7/10 of one second.

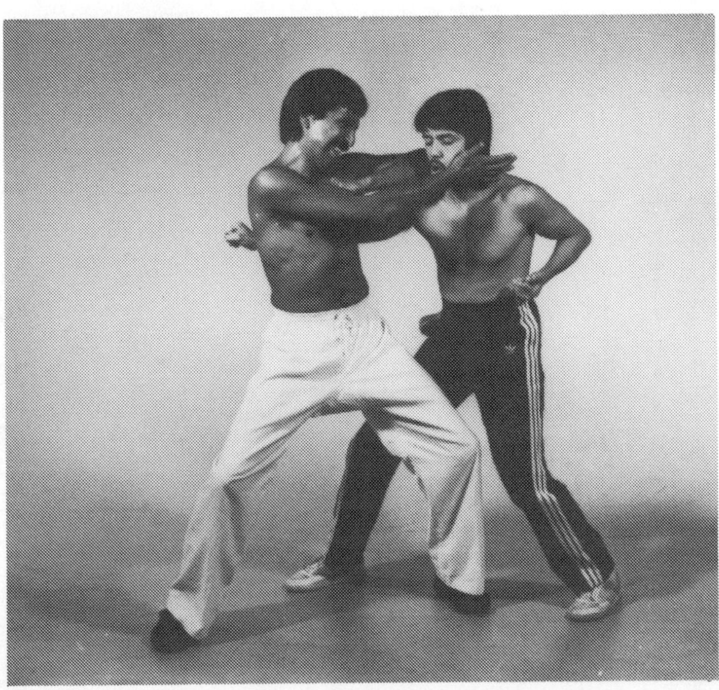

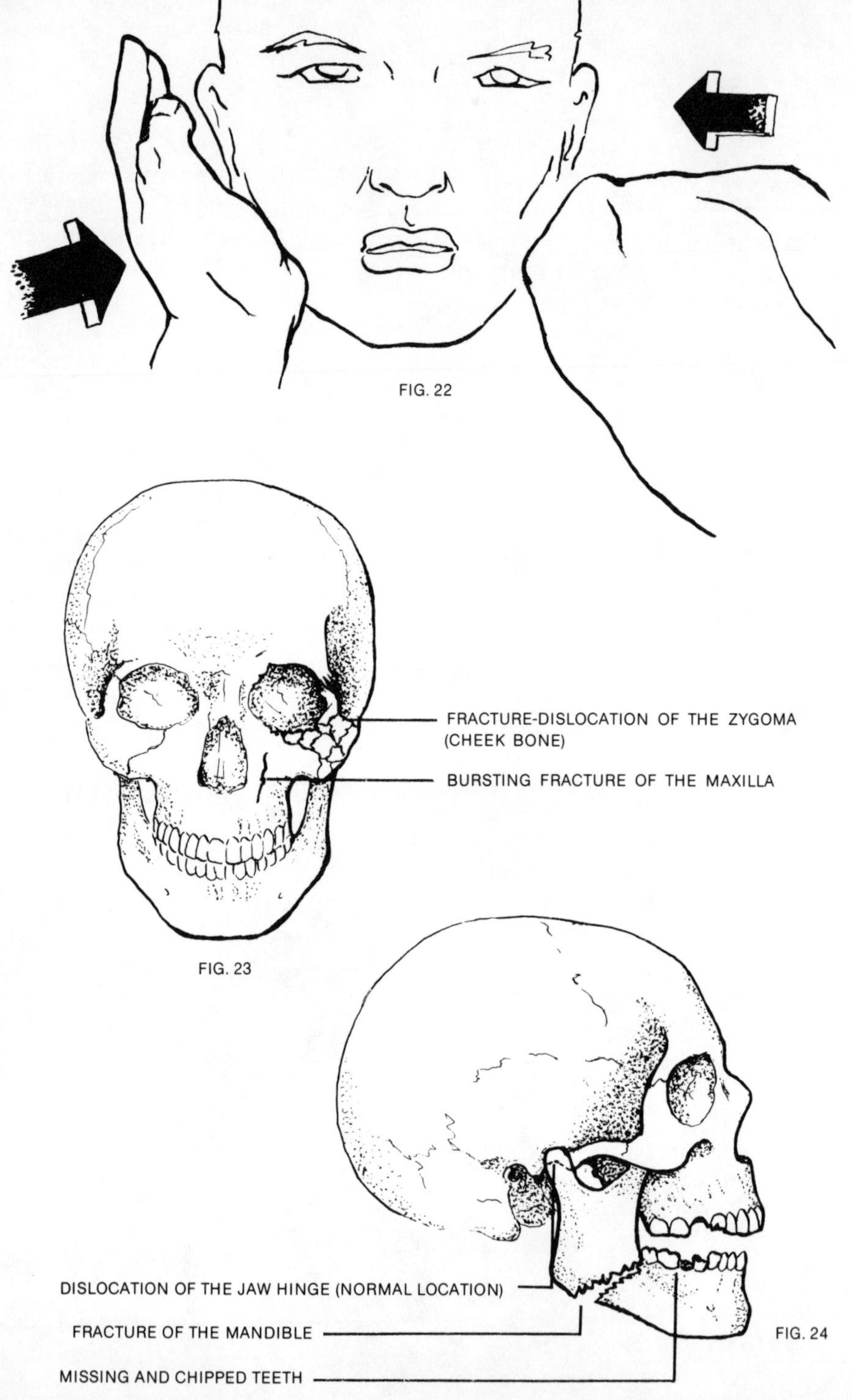

FIG. 22

FIG. 23

FIG. 24

WEAPON: Elbow and Palm strike
TARGET: Jaw

Medical Implications

I. A FRACTURE OR DISLOCATION OF THE MANDIBLE (lower jaw) is a very apparent result of two striking surfaces on either side of the jawbone. If both strikes were simultaneous, a double fracture (one on each side) would be evident. But if one weapon were to arrive before the other, thus pushing the jaw into the path of the other weapon, then only a fracture on one side would be applicable. In order to prevent a future deformity of the jaw line, the teeth and fragments must be temporarily wired together. Of course there will be great difficulty eating and speaking until complete healing has taken place. Dislocation of the jaw hinge would easily occur if the blow were near the upper portion of the jaw and were a glancing type blow. The wider the opening of the mouth at the moment of impact, the easier it would be for the dislocation to occur.

II. A FRACTURE DISLOCATION OF THE ZYGOMA (cheekbone) would result if the elbow struck a short distance above the jaw. A bursting fracture in the bone surrounding the cheekbone may result from the crushing pressure of the elbow. The maxillary sinus lies under the cheekbone and would undoubtedly be lacerated by bone fragments from the fracture. Blood would fill the sinus and flow into the throat or out of the nose. The possibilities of unconsciousness and concussion range very high. (Refer to Chapter 1.)

III. THE FACIAL NERVE MAY BE PINCHED OR ABRADED against the edge of the mandible and (according to how devastating the damage) may leave part or all of one side of the face in paralysis (Fig. 8).

IV. CONTROL OF THE TONGUE WOULD BE LOST because of the mandible fracture. Torn muscles on the bottom of the mouth that adhere the tongue would go into spasm and if unconsciousness ensued, the tongue along with the broken and dislocated teeth would be swallowed and death by choking would follow.

8
Striking the Throat

Against a knife thrust to the throat, defender sidesteps as he parries the thrust across his body with his left hand.

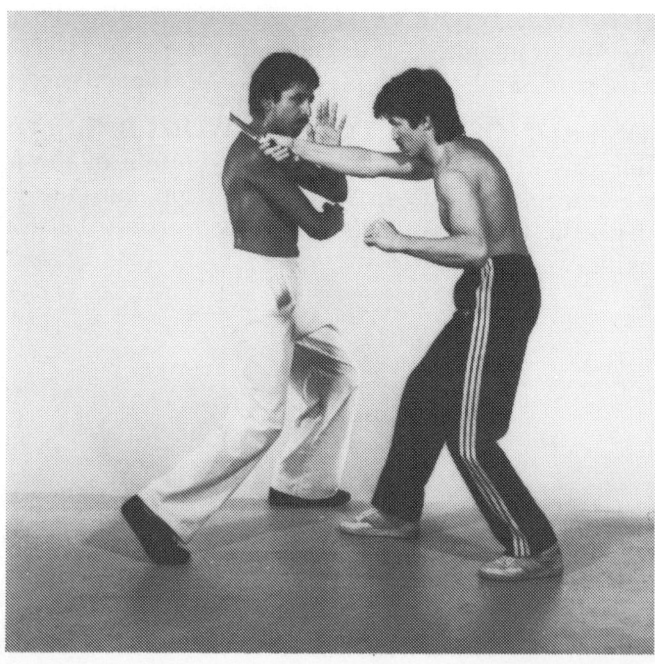

The right hand grabs attacker's wrist, pulls him forward as defender prepares to strike to the throat.

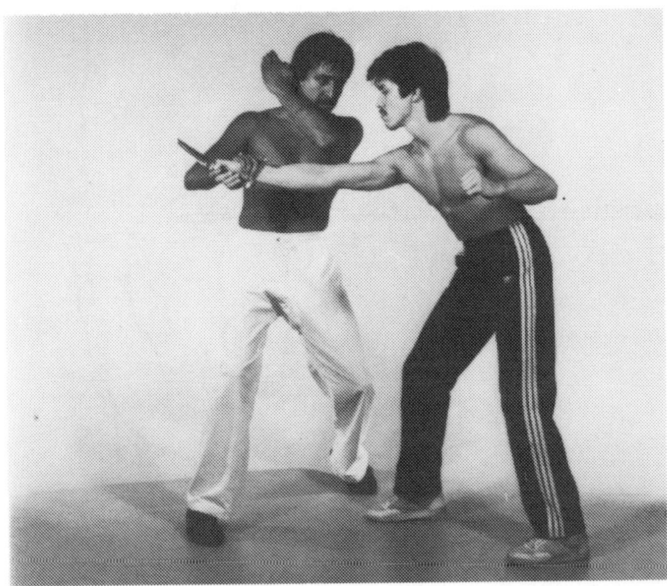

Defender jerks opponent's arm, jerking the head back, exposing the throat and strikes. This technique was completed in 6/10 of one second.

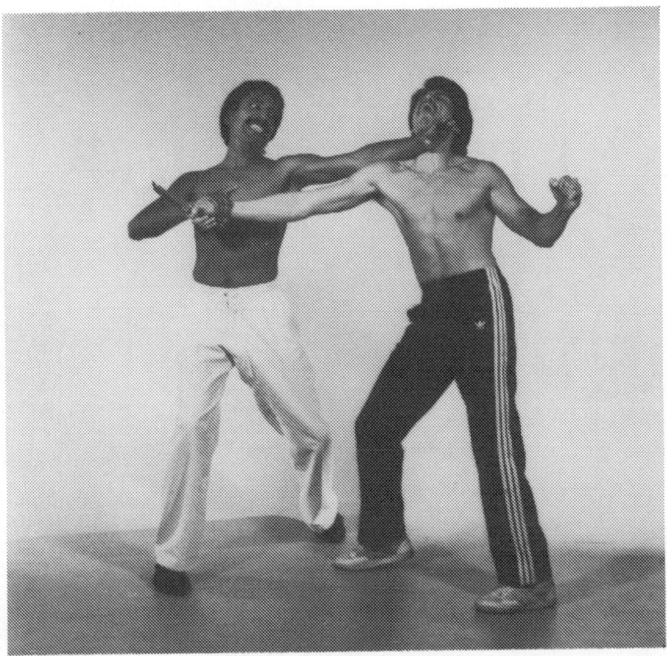

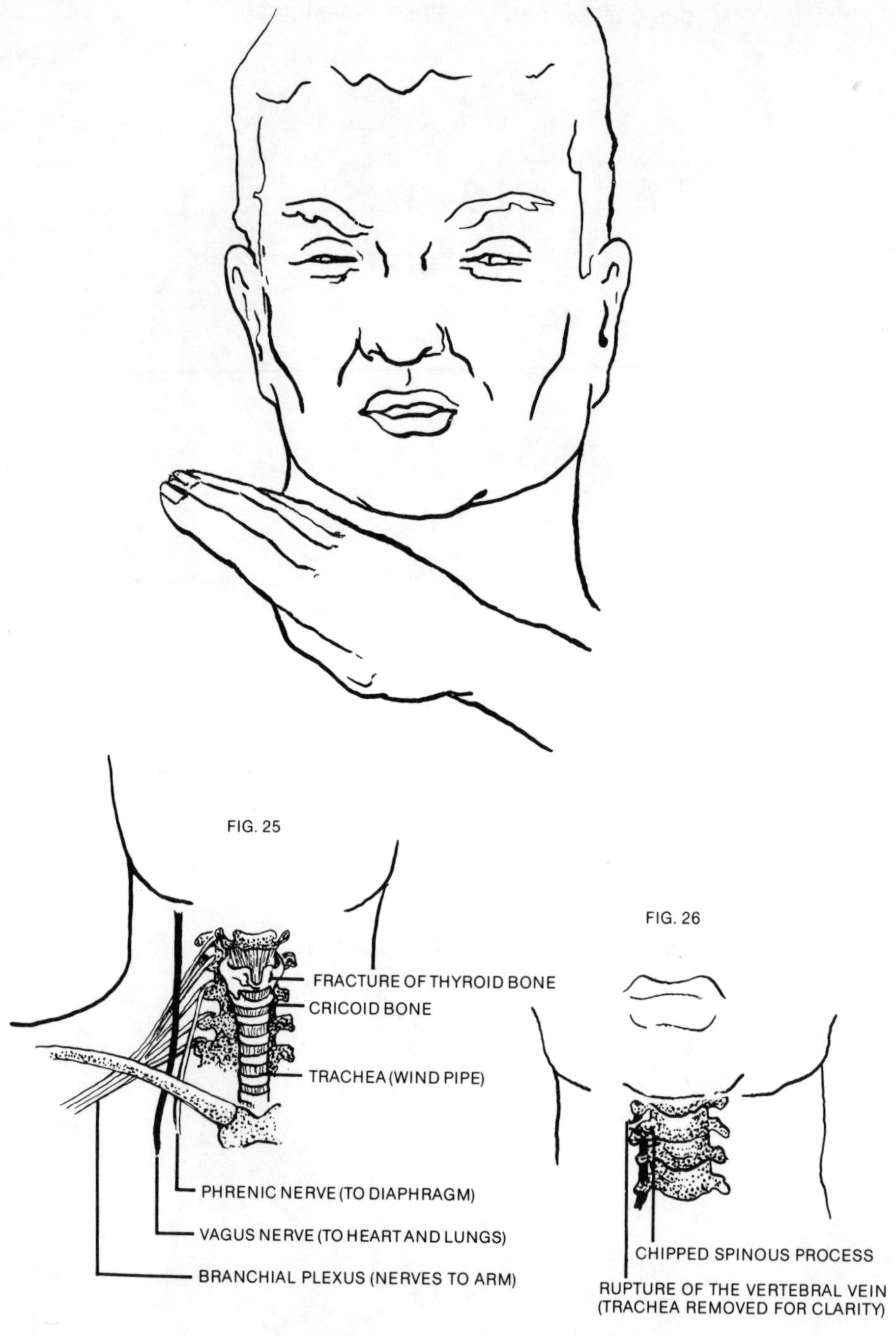
FIG. 25
FRACTURE OF THYROID BONE
CRICOID BONE
TRACHEA (WIND PIPE)
PHRENIC NERVE (TO DIAPHRAGM)
VAGUS NERVE (TO HEART AND LUNGS)
BRANCHIAL PLEXUS (NERVES TO ARM)
FIG. 26
CHIPPED SPINOUS PROCESS
RUPTURE OF THE VERTEBRAL VEIN
(TRACHEA REMOVED FOR CLARITY)

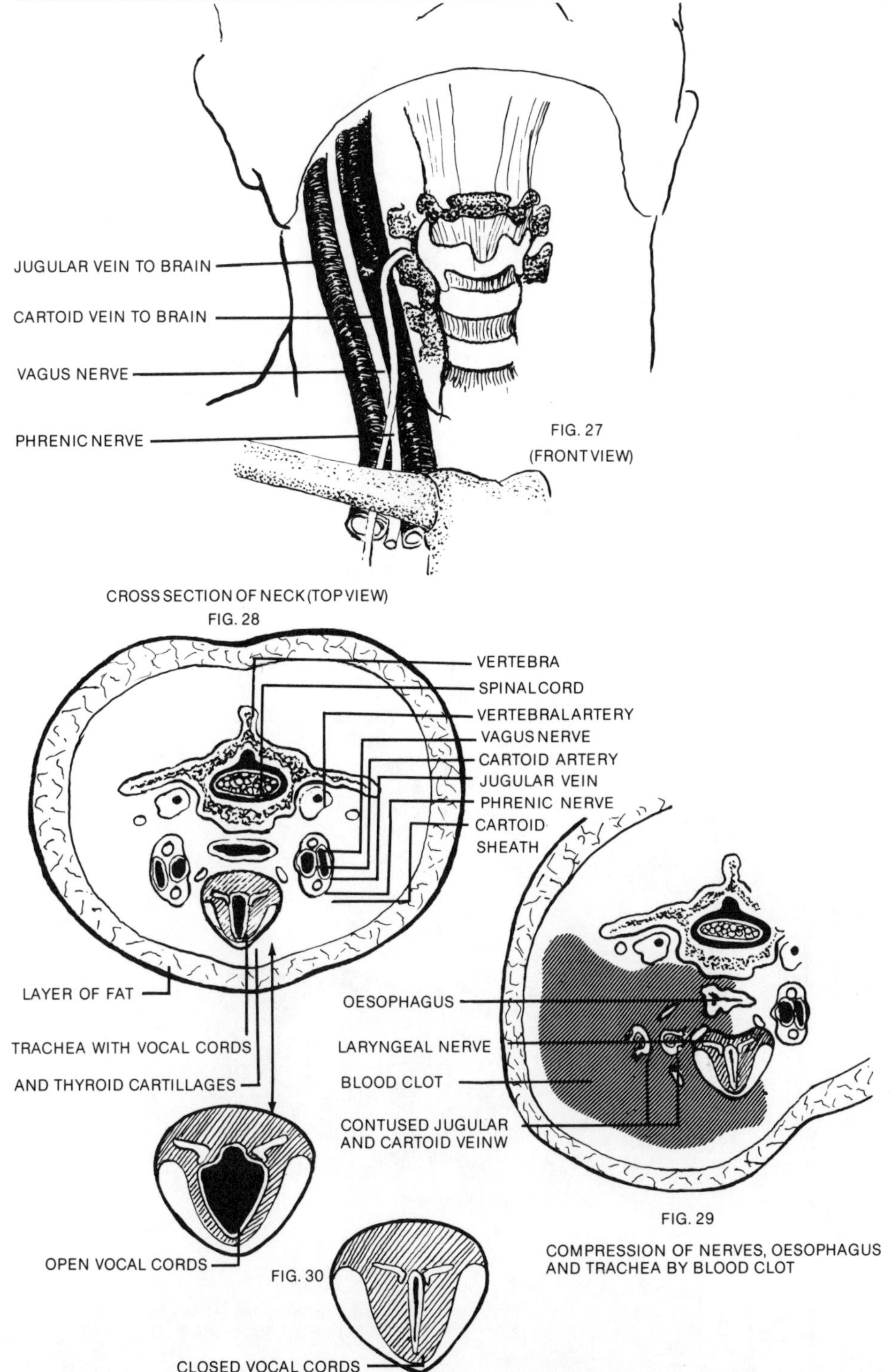
JUGULAR VEIN TO BRAIN
CARTOID VEIN TO BRAIN
VAGUS NERVE
PHRENIC NERVE
FIG. 27
(FRONT VIEW)
CROSS SECTION OF NECK (TOP VIEW)
FIG. 28
VERTEBRA
SPINAL CORD
VERTEBRAL ARTERY
VAGUS NERVE
CARTOID ARTERY
JUGULAR VEIN
PHRENIC NERVE
CARTOID SHEATH
LAYER OF FAT
TRACHEA WITH VOCAL CORDS
AND THYROID CARTILLAGES
OESOPHAGUS
LARYNGEAL NERVE
BLOOD CLOT
CONTUSED JUGULAR
AND CARTOID VEINW
FIG. 29
COMPRESSION OF NERVES, OESOPHAGUS
AND TRACHEA BY BLOOD CLOT
OPEN VOCAL CORDS
FIG. 30
CLOSED VOCAL CORDS

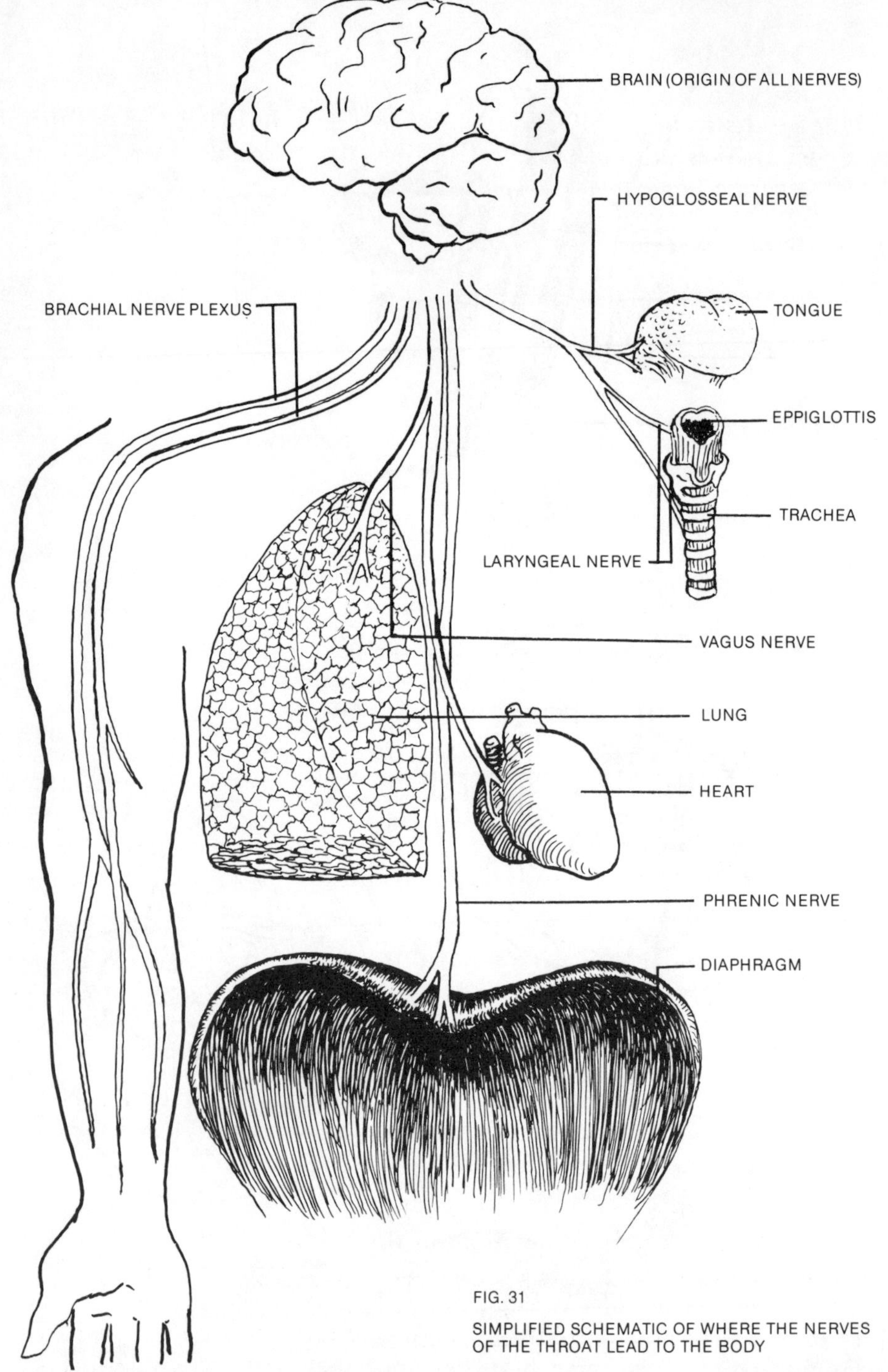

FIG. 31

SIMPLIFIED SCHEMATIC OF WHERE THE NERVES OF THE THROAT LEAD TO THE BODY

WEAPON: Chop (Side of the hand)
TARGET: Side or front of the throat

Medical Implications

The results from a well-focused blow to the front or side of the throat are a combination of multiple effects and results. The following is a listing of each separate possible effect and result:

Effects

(1) Contusion of the internal *Jugular Vein*
(2) Contusion of the internal *Carotid Vein*
(3) Contusion of the *Vertebratal Vein*
(4) Contusion of the *Hypoglassal Nerve*
(5) Contusion of the *Vagus Nerve*
(6) Contusion of the *Phrenic Nerve*
(7) Contusion of the *Laryngenial Nerve*
(8) Hematoma in *Carotid Sheath*
(9) Fracture of the *Spinous Process*
(10) Fracture of the *Thyroid Cartilage*
(11) Fracture of the *Cricoid Cartilage*
(12) Possible injury to *Branchial Plexus* (Refer to Chapter 10.)

Results

I. The internal jugular vein pulsates during respiration, distends during expiration, and collapses to a ribbon-like structure during inspiration. If the blow struck on expiration, the vein would be full of blood and hard. Rupturing of the internal jugular vein from striking it against the hard surface of the cervical vertebra would result in a quick death due to a massive hemorrhage (hematoma).

II. Severe contusion of the carotid vein may result in thrombosis, (blood clot in the vessel) due to the vessel wall spasm, which produces a restriction in blood flow. This may eventually end in cerebral thrombosis (blood clot in vessels of the brain) and death.

III. Laceration or contusion of the VERTEBRAL ARTERY is only possible when the blow is heavy enough to chip or fracture the spinous vertebral processes that the artery runs through. Results are the same as the previous two variations in vessel damage.

IV. The two most important functions of the VAGUS NERVE we are concerned with here are that of heart contraction and lung constriction. Since there are two branches of the vagus nerve (one on each side of the neck) injury to one may not by itself be completely fatal because of the partial overlapping of the two nerve branches once they reach their destination.

However, damage to one side of the nerve could cause spasms of the lungs and heart, ultimately ending in shortness of breath, irregular heart palputations, and death.

V. The PHRENIC NERVE runs from the fourth cervical vertebra, vertically down the neck into the thorax (chest) where it finally merges into the diaphram. The main function of the phrenic nerve is to supply the diaphram with necessary responses for breathing. When it is injured, the same feeling that one gets when the "wind" has been knocked out will exist until normal function resumes or death occurs.

VI. The LARYNGEAL NERVES (nerves of the vocal cords, etc.) are a branch of the vagus nerve. They control the main functions of the larynx, which are to open and close the vocal cords and epiglottis so that no foreign objects are permitted to pass through the trachea. When a foreign object (food, teeth, blood, etc.) agitates the nerve surrounding the larynx or inside of the throat, the vocal cords close and the epiglottis covers the opening of the wind pipe to prevent anything from being sucked into the pipe. When this is done no air can go in or out of the lungs until the nerve relaxes and opens the wind pipe for normal breathing. If the nerve does not relax, death by suffocation will follow.

VII. The HYPOGLOSSAL NERVE is the main nerve of the tongue. If it is damaged, loss of control of the tongue will be inevitable with suffocation and death if it is swallowed.

VIII. A HEMATOMA IN THE SHEATH that encompasses the internal jugular, carotid vein and vagus nerve in the neck is the result of blood leakage from a torn blood vessel.

If the tear does not seal itself immediately, death by strangulation will soon follow. The hematoma will grow larger with each pulsation of the heart and eventually start pressing against the trachea until it has compressed it enough to stimulate the laryngeal nerves to close it off. The outside appearance will be that of a huge swelling on the side of the neck (Fig. 29).

IX. A chipped or fractured SPINOUS PROCESS of the vertebra is one of the most dangerous occurances, not because of the fracture but because of what lies between it and the outside surface of the skin, which in this case is everything previously mentioned in this Chapter. Also there would be the possibility of spinal cord shock (injury to the spinal cord without any known disruption of the spinal cord fibers—*whiplash*).

X. Fracture of the THYROID OR CRICOID CARTILAGE is the result of a frontal blow to the throat. The most important thing to remember here is that surrounding the cartilages are many nerve branches of the larynx (laryngenial nerves). Of course, stimulation of these nerves by a fracture of the cartilage will activate the vocal cords and epiglottis to close off the air supply to the lungs, resulting in a slow death by suffocation or at least unconsciousness from lack of air.

Because of the close proximity of all the above mentioned effects and results, it is easy to see how two or more of the effects would exist and cause death to or at least total disability of the attacker.

9
Striking the Back of the Neck

Against an overhead club strike, defender sidesteps as his left arm parries the blow downward. The right arm is cocked for counterattack.

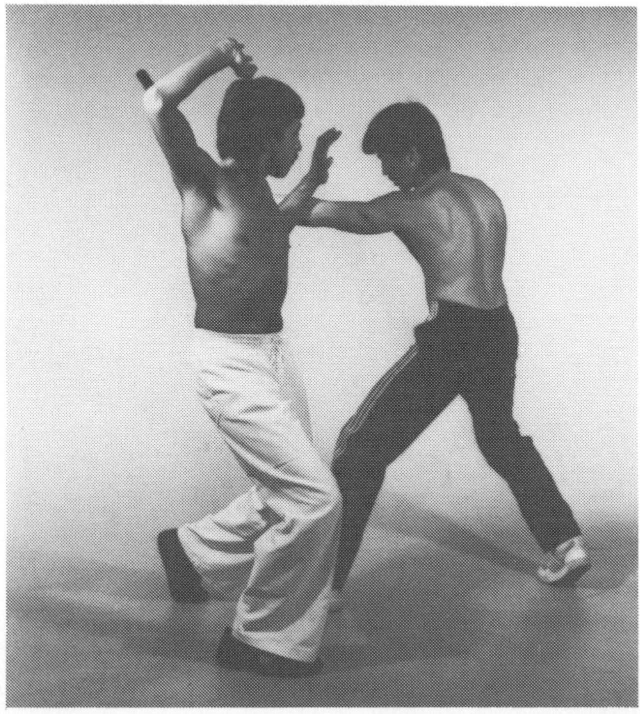

Defender strikes to the back of the neck as he pulls opponent's arm, pivoting to add momentum to the strike. This technique was completed in 7/10 of one second.

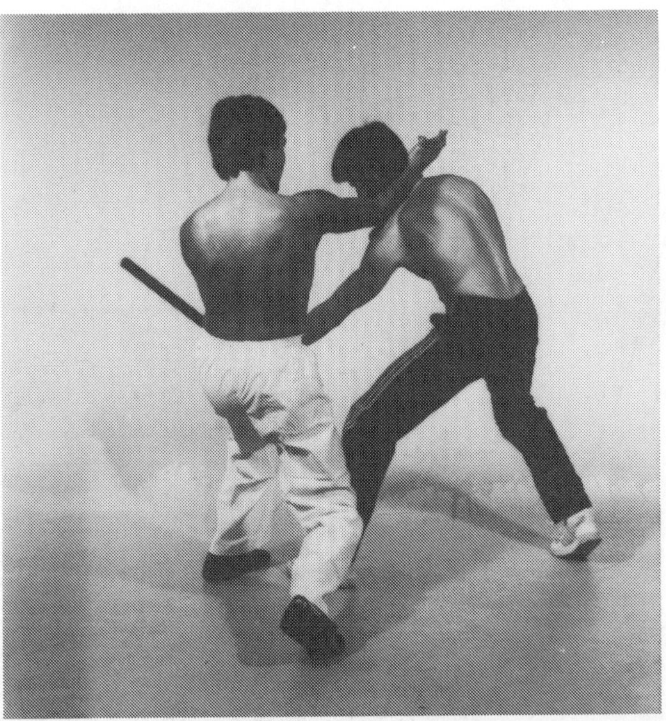

CONCUSSIVE VIBRATION

FIG. 32

SPINAL CORD

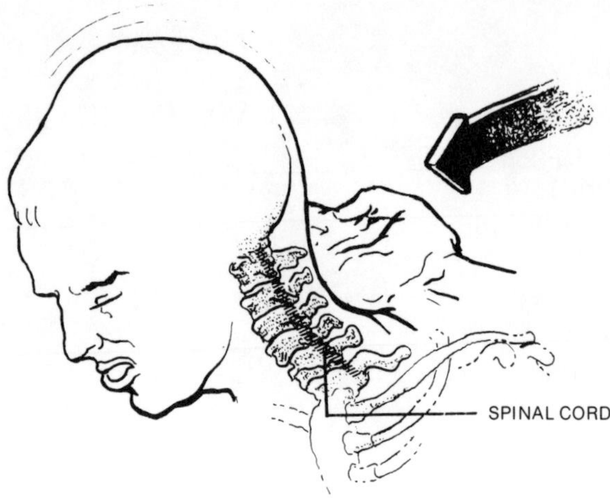

CUT-AWAY THROUGH MIDDLE OF SPINAL COLUMN

FIG. 33

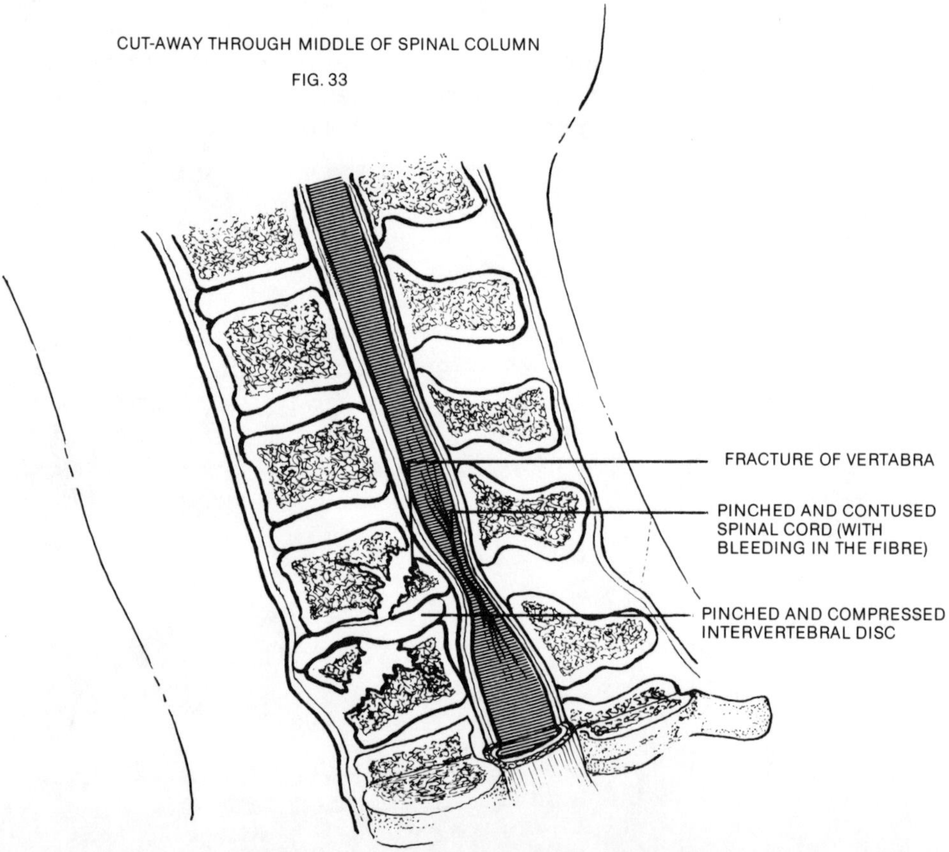

FRACTURE OF VERTABRA
PINCHED AND CONTUSED SPINAL CORD (WITH BLEEDING IN THE FIBRE)
PINCHED AND COMPRESSED INTERVERTEBRAL DISC

WEAPON: Chop (Side of the hand)
TARGET: Back of the neck

Medical Implications

I. Muscle spasms and a WHIPLASH INJURY should be considered the minimum possible damage resulting from this type of blow. There is also a possibility that the blow might result in permanent spinal cord shock (injury to the spinal cord—better known as a whiplash injury). Noticeable symptoms will appear immediately or at a later date. These symptoms occur in many degrees of severity, from constant neck strain (as if a muscle were pulled) and severe headaches, to pains throughout the neck and back area.

II. A broken neck is the term used to specify a SEVERED SPINAL CORD. This is usually accomplished by the severing action of a fractured vertebra. Complete paralysis from the point of impact downward will result.

If the cord is severed above the fifth cervical vertebra, death will be immediate.

The spinal cord is very much like a multiple strand telephone cable in the sense that it is composed of many nerve strands, and these strands together make up one dense cord. The phrenic nerve is most accessible between the second and fourth vertebrae. If it is severed it will be fatal, because it controls the function of the diaphragm in breathing. Shock, loss of consciousness, coma, and death waste no time in arriving.

III. Multiple FRACTURE OF THE CERVICAL VERTEBRA with bleeding in a pinched spinal cord will cause partial to complete paralysis encompassing any or all portions of the body and limbs below the point of impact. Respiratory paralysis may be due to a compressed phrenic nerve. Death may be immediate or occur later. Inability to move the head from side to side, dizziness and headache are the minimal possibilities from a medium-strength blow.

A CONCUSSION may exist due to the transmission of shock waves through the brain stem into the brain. Shock (caused by too much stress on the nervous system) may by itself cause death. This is sometimes referred to as a violent interruption of the body's homostatic balance.

10

Striking the Collar Bone

Against a one arm palm push, the defender steps to the outside, parries the push with his left forearm, and cocks his right arm in preparation for the strike.

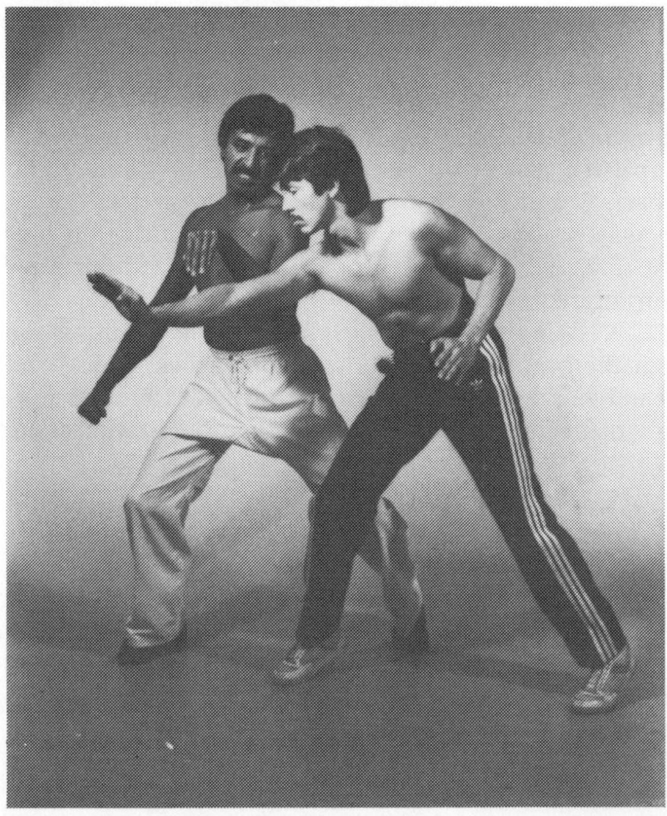

The defender pulls the attacker's arm downward with a hooking motion as he steps behind the attacker's forward leg, and swings his right arm in an overhead circle to deliver an elbow blow to the attacker's collarbone. This technique was completed in 8/10 of one second.

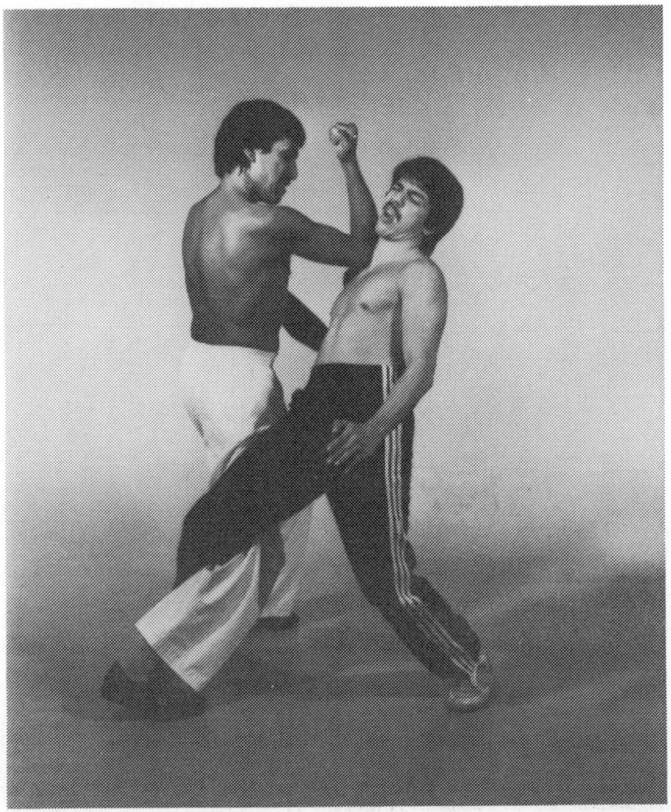

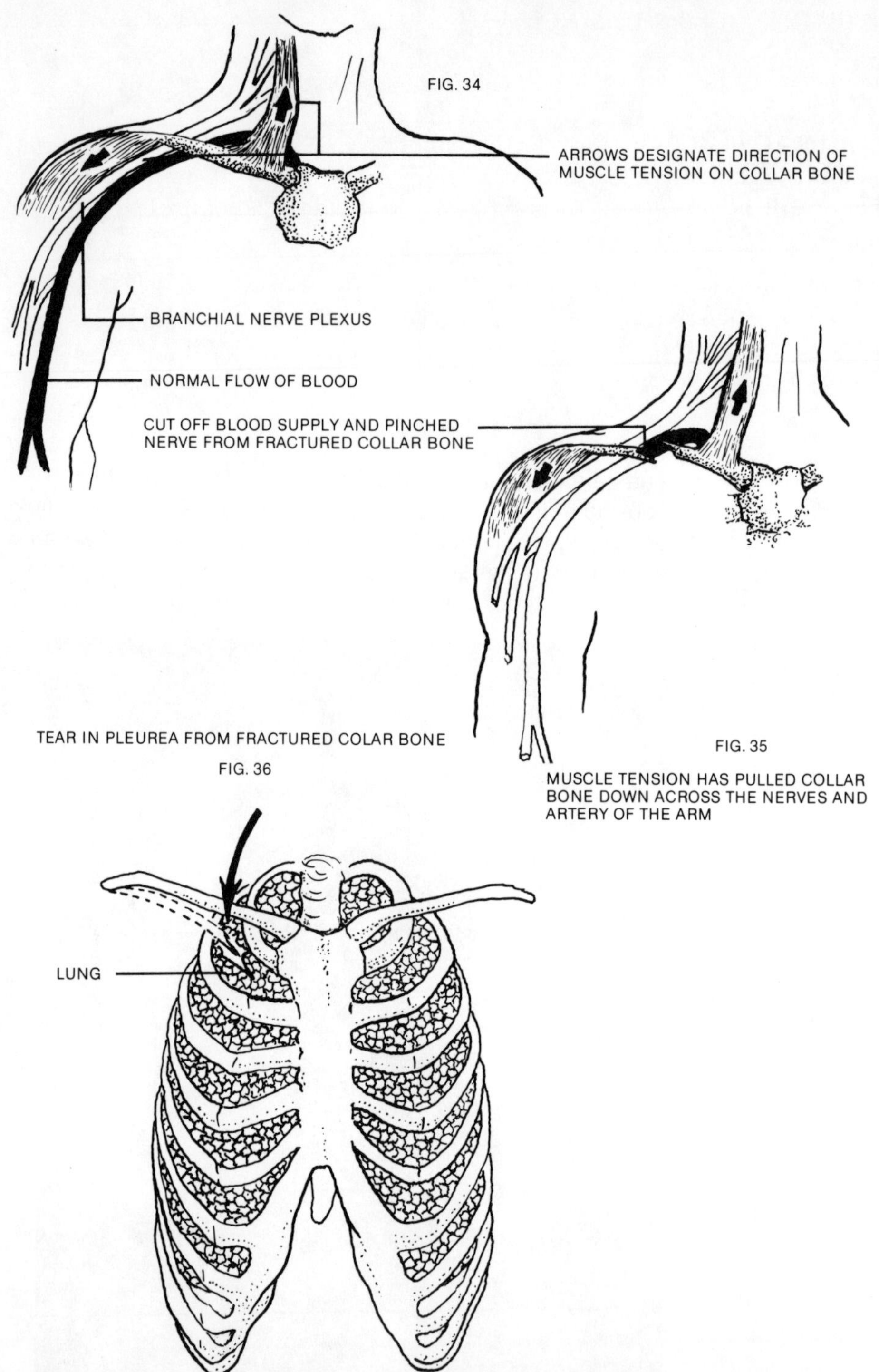
FIG. 34
ARROWS DESIGNATE DIRECTION OF
MUSCLE TENSION ON COLLAR BONE
BRANCHIAL NERVE PLEXUS
NORMAL FLOW OF BLOOD
CUT OFF BLOOD SUPPLY AND PINCHED
NERVE FROM FRACTURED COLLAR BONE
FIG. 35
MUSCLE TENSION HAS PULLED COLLAR
BONE DOWN ACROSS THE NERVES AND
ARTERY OF THE ARM
TEAR IN PLEUREA FROM FRACTURED COLAR BONE
FIG. 36
LUNG

WEAPON: Elbow
TARGET: Collar Bone (Clavicle)

Medical Implications

I. A FRACTURE OF THE COLLAR BONE (CLAVICLE) would surely disable the opponent's arm on the side of the body the fracture was on. There will be an obvious dropping of the shoulder accompanied by sharp pains.

II. Common complications of the fracture are severance or LACERATION OF THE BRANCHIAL NERVE PLEXUS AND SUBCLAVIAN ARTERY. Severance or laceration of the branchial nerve will cause paralysis of part or all of the arm. Laceration of the artery is also a common side effect because it follows the nerve closely (under the collar bone, Fig. 34). If the artery was merely pinched (due to muscle tension pulling up and down on the collar bone—Fig. 35) and blood was not allowed to pursue it's normal path through the arm, thrombosis* would occur. The pinched artery must be remedied within four to six hours or the risk of gangrene will be present.

III. If the blow is a heavy one, it can push the jagged edge of the broken bone down far enough to reach the lung. The sharp edges of the break will puncture the plurae (thin sac-like membrane covering the lung) and the lung will gradually deflate. Shortness of breath, air starvation, painful breathing, dizzyness, irregular heart palpitations, unconsciousness, coma and death are the general symptoms of a collapsed lung (Chapter 12, Fig. 42).

* Thrombosis: A Blood clot in the artery, restricting normal flow of blood.)

11

Striking the Solar Plexus

Attacker grabs both of the defender's wrists from behind.

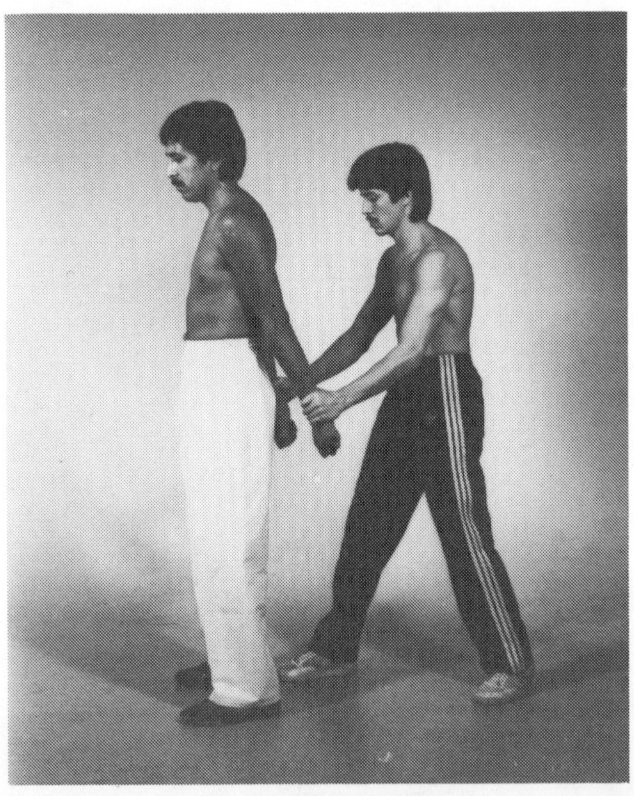

Defender steps forward, pulling attacker's body forward and off-balance. Defender simultaneously countergrabs attacker's wrists.

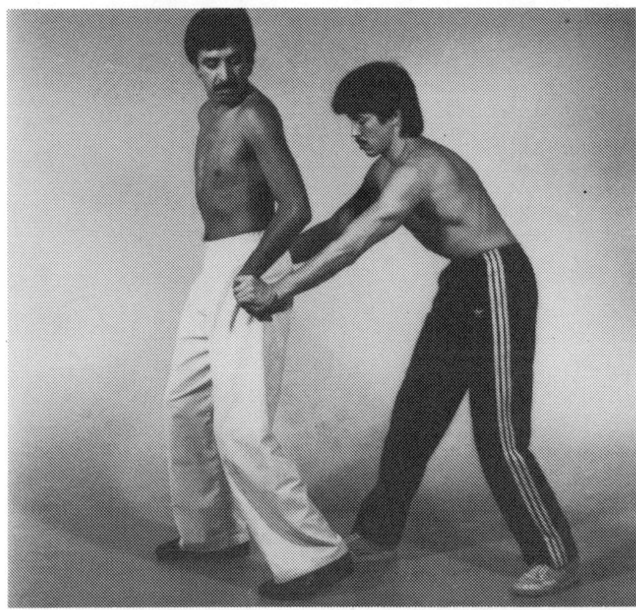

Defender delivers backkick to attacker's abdomen, making contact with his heel. This technique was completed in 7/10 of one second.

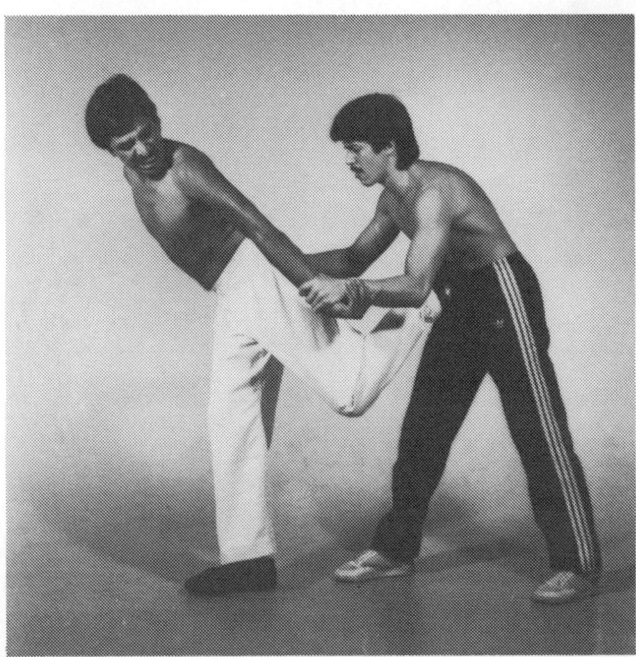

FIG. 37

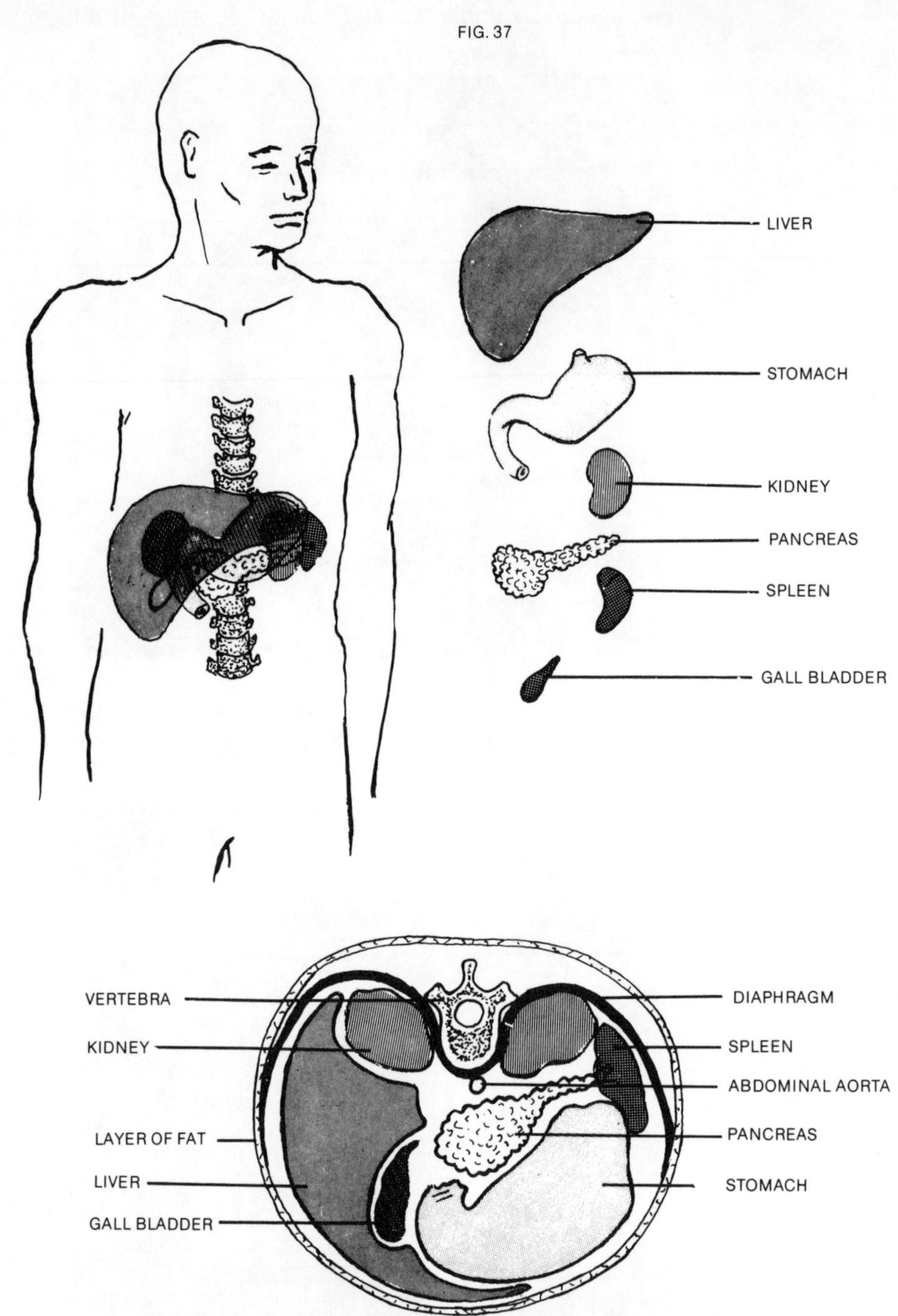

TOP VIEW OF SOLAR PLEXUS (CUT-AWAY)

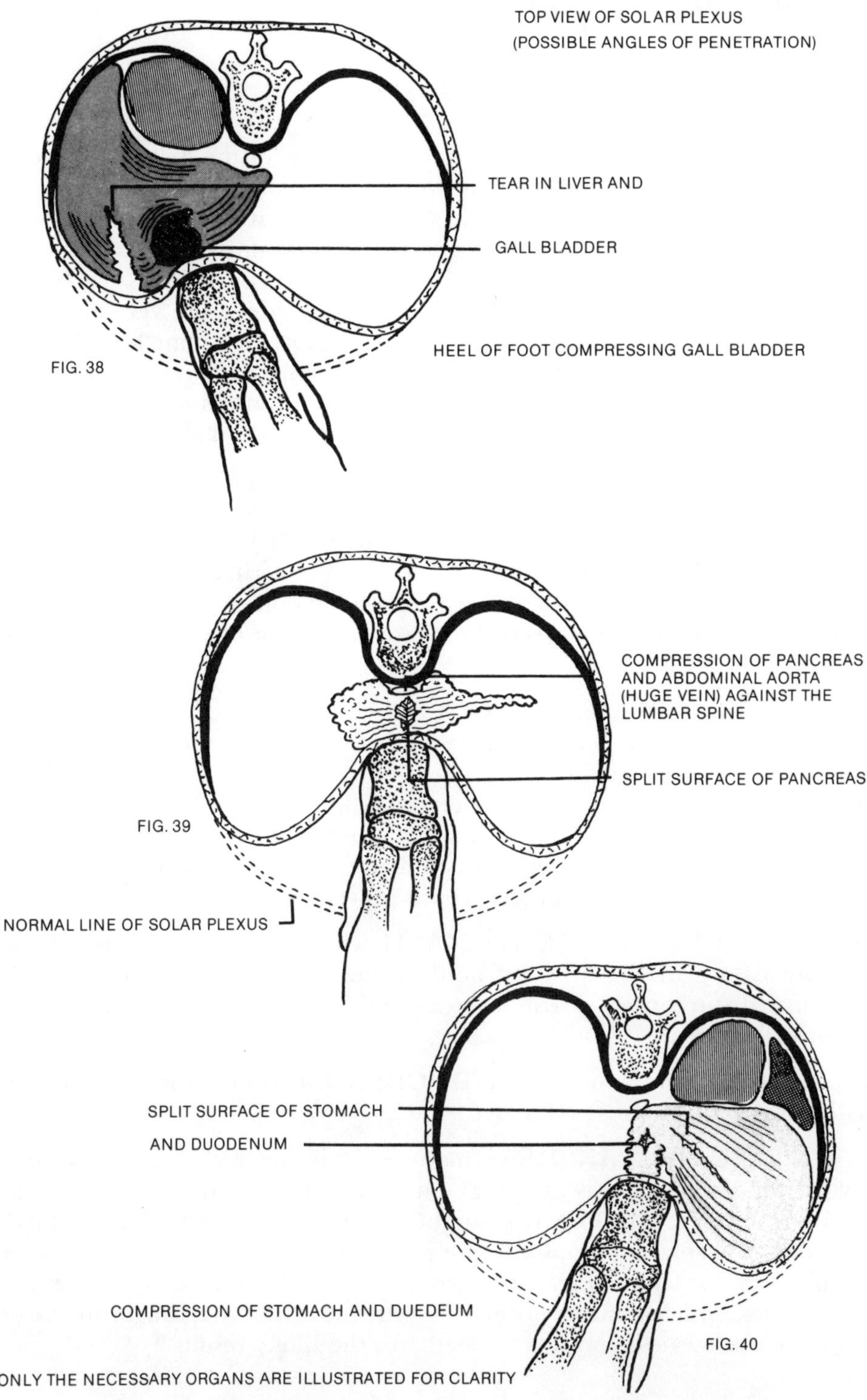

*ONLY THE NECESSARY ORGANS ARE ILLUSTRATED FOR CLARITY

WEAPON: Heel of the foot
TARGET: Solar Plexus

Medical Implications

As indicated in Figures 38, 39, 40, different angles of the kick will produce varied results. If the kick is directed toward the right side of the opponent's body, the liver and gallbladder will be damaged. If it is in the center of the solar plexus, the duodenum and pancreas will be thrust against the front of the lumbar spine. The abdominal aorta (huge vein) follows the lumbar spine vertically and is very snug against the front side of the vertebra. If the heel kick was strong enough to injure the vein, shock (extreme loss of blood) and death would follow almost immediately. The stomach (and some reports claim that the spleen) will be involved when the blow is to the left side of the solar plexus. The level, angle and strength of the kick will determine how many of these organs will be damaged.

I. A DEEP FISSURE IN THE LIVER may very well be fatal. Peritonitis in the name given to free floating blood and/or bile in the peritoneal cavity (body cavity). Hiccupping from blood or bile irritating the diaphragm and an increasing tenderness and pain in the abdomen will continue until surgery of the abdomen corrects the symptoms which may very easily evolve into death.

II. THE GALL BLADDER WOULD BE TORN with gastric acids and digestive juices being spilled into the body cavity. (Prior to a meal, the gall bladder fills with proper digestive juices for digestion of the meal and stores the juices until food is induced. The gall bladder would burst rather easily if enough pressure was exerted upon it during the predigestion period.) The juices would immediately start to digest the internal organs they came in contact with, and only surgery would prevent death.

III. RUPTURE OF THE STOMACH with the spilling of its contents and blood into the body cavity would again result in peritonitis. Days of intestinal disturbances, gastric disorders and vomiting, shock, and eventual death will occur.

IV. A compression injury of the DUODENUM against the lumbar spine will progress the same as III above.

V. AN INJURED PANCREAS may result if the kick were well timed (when the opponent was inhaling) and the solar plexus were relaxed and easily penetrated. The pancreas might also be compressed, along with the duodenum, against the lumbar spine producing a split surface of the organ. Respiratory paralysis (Fig. 45)—spasm of the abdominal and intercostal rib muscles, which inhibits normal movements of the diaphragm in breathing—unconsciousness, shock, and death are the likely results.

VI. PARTIAL COLLAPSE OF THE LUNG (refer to Chapter 12), due to a minute plural tear from the percussive shock (jarring) present in the chest cavity at the moment of impact, will result in shallow breathing and great pain during respiration.

VII. SHOCK is a term used in internal injuries to describe the extreme loss of blood and bile into the body cavity. Shock may be immediately fatal or be latent (48 hours later) until abdominal splinting occurs. Abdominal splinting means that when the cavity fills with blood, it will be evident because of a growing tenderness and increasing rididity of the abdomen, with the elevation of body temperature and possible vomiting of blood from rupture of the stomach or duodenum. Death is the common result of shock, because usually by the time the injured person arrives at the hospital he has lapsed into unconsciousness from lack of blood and cannot tell the doctor his symptoms.

12
Striking the Side of the Rib Cage

Against a left jab, defender steps back and slightly to the outside as he parries the punch and prepares to counter.

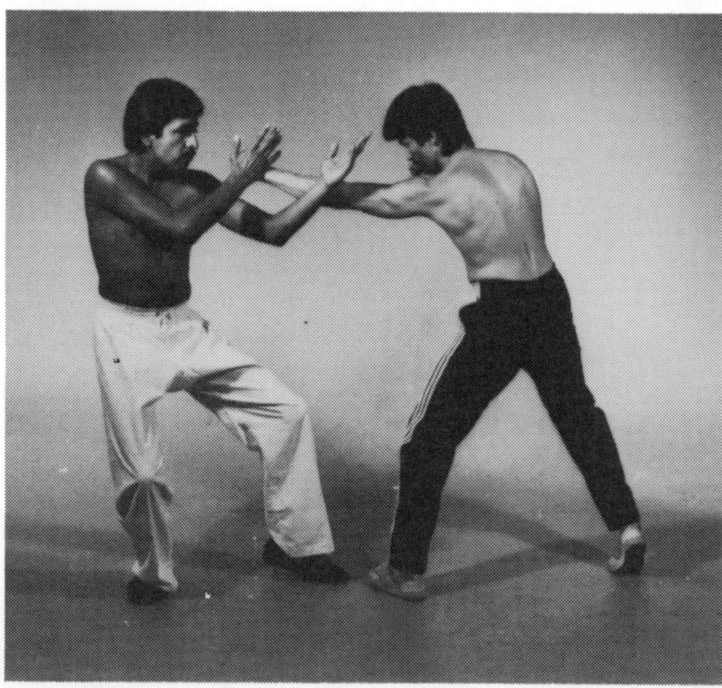

Defender grabs attacker's left wrist, pulls the arm toward him, exposing attacker's ribcage. He pivots on his right leg and strikes ribcage with his heel. This technique was completed in 8/10 of one second.

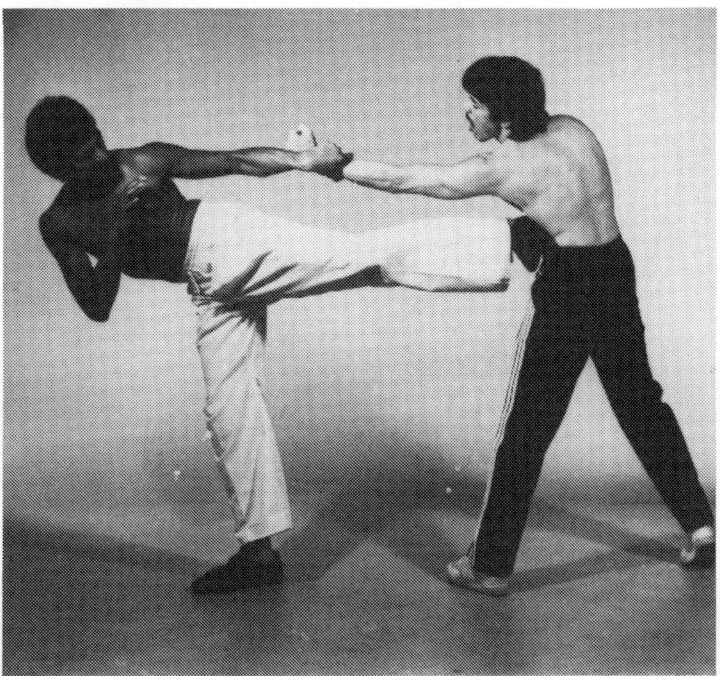

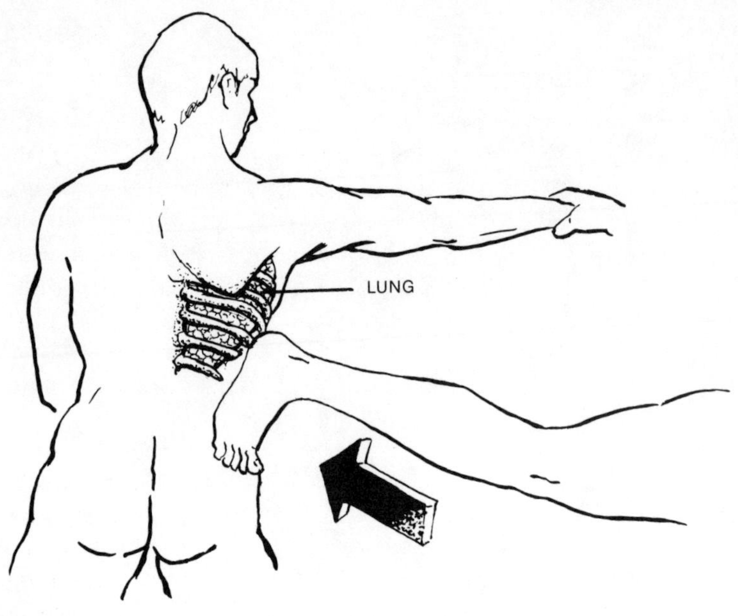

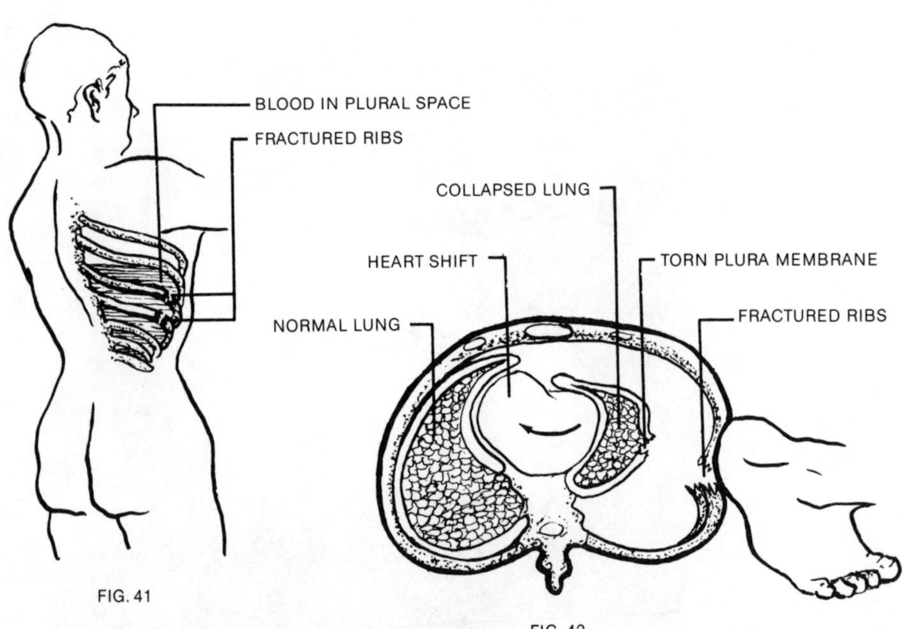

FIG. 41

FIG. 42
TOP VIEW (CUT-AWAY)

WEAPON: Heel of foot
TARGET: Side of ribs

Medical Implications

I. A green stick fracture* of the ribs will cause only pain in breathing, but a complete break in the rib, with protruding ends, will tear the lung's pleura (membrane sac covering the lungs) and puncture the lung, resulting in a COLLAPSED LUNG. Blood in the lung cavity (hemothorax) will be present until it is removed. Shortness of breath and muscle spasms of the chest and rib cage, with severe pain while breathing will predominate. If the lung collapses all the way, death is sure to follow. A lung may be collapsed from the violent jarring produced by the kick, without the presence of a fractured rib. When the pleura tear is very small, it will usually seal itself soon without any great after effects.

The great danger involved with a completely collapsed lung (besides air starvation) is an uncontrollable spasm of the heart, which is caused by the pressure difference when the lung collapses. The heart is held in place (partially) by the lungs on either side and the heart's suspensory ligaments. When there is no pressure on one side to help hold the heart in place, the lung on the other side will pull the heart toward it (heart shift), resulting in a severe muscle spasm of the heart and usually either a quick or lingering death. Intercostal muscle spasms (muscles between the ribs) with loss of breath would be the minimal damage (refer to Chapter 13, Fig. 45). A complication of this blow would be a puncture of the diaphragm (refer to Chapter 13, Fig. 46).

* A green stick fracture is when the fracture line runs down the middle of the bone, but does not completely break the continuity of the bone.

13
Striking the Diaphragm

Against a headlock, defender moves into a sidestance. His left hand reaches for the attacker's face while his right arm cocks for the strike.

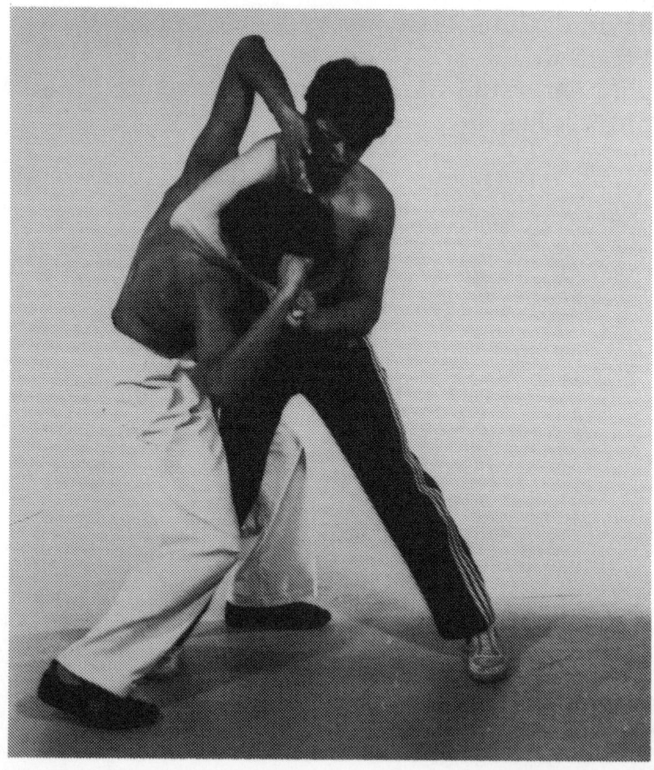

The defender pushes up under attacker's nose, forcing his head back.

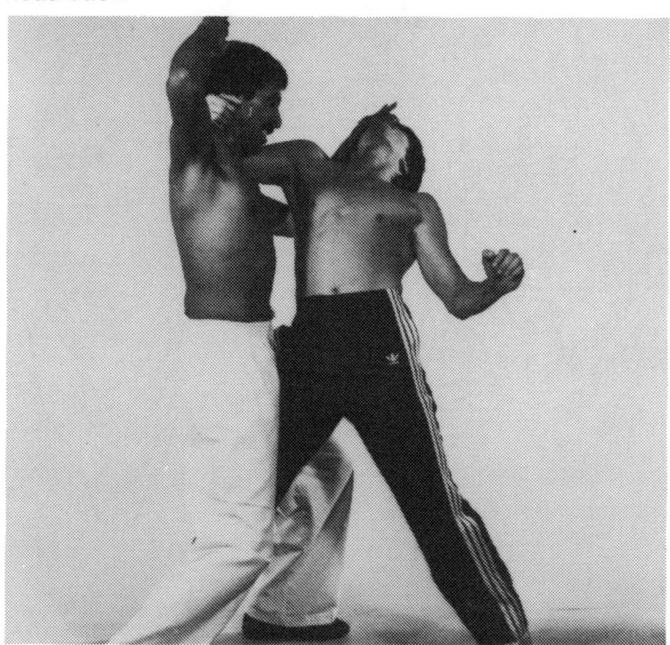

Defender strikes to the exposed diaphragm with a hammerfist, the blow directed to either side of the sternum. This technique was completed in 7/10 of one second.

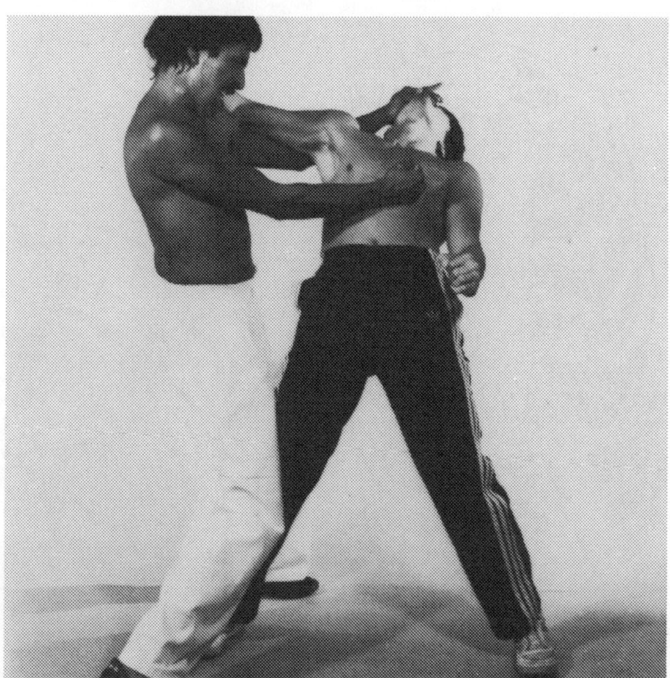

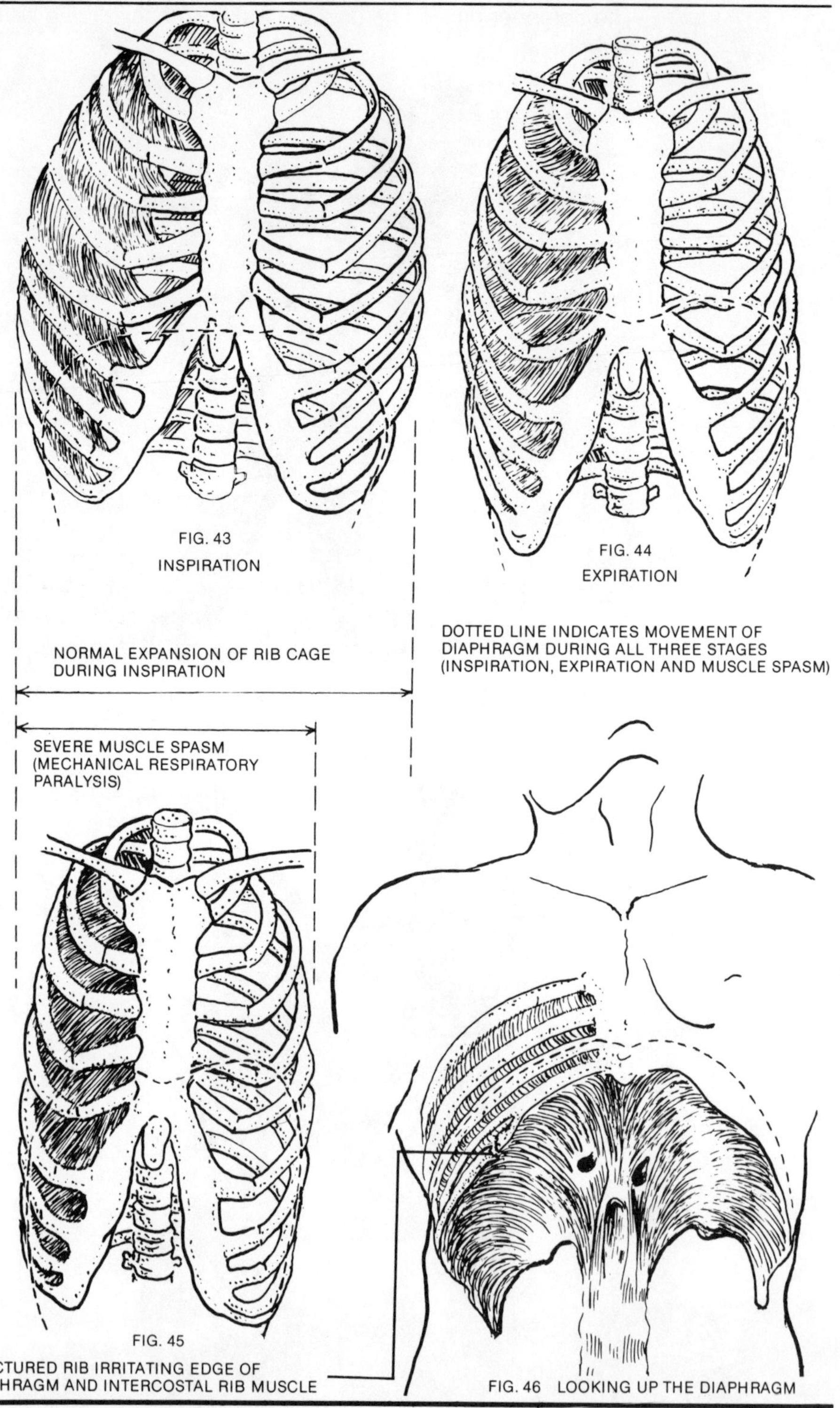

FIG. 43
INSPIRATION

FIG. 44
EXPIRATION

FIG. 45

FIG. 46 LOOKING UP THE DIAPHRAGM

WEAPON: Hammerfist
TARGET: Diaphragm

Medical Implications

I. Just a light tap near the lower frontal ribs will cause a slight contraction of the diaphragm and intercostal muscles. The diaphragm's main function is that of respiration. The intercostal muscles (muscles between each rib) take over the function of the diaphragm in situations of stress, but they soon tire and will not function properly. A hard blow to the diaphragm or ribs will relax those muscles and all breathing will cease for the moment because when relaxed, the muscles force the air out of the lungs and continue to squeeze until the muscles let the ribs expand again for inspiration of air. Unconsciousness, due to a mechanical respiratory paralysis (Fig. 45), is a common result from such a blow.

II. The jagged edge of a fractured rib irritating the surface of the diaphragm will produce "shallow breathing." The diaphragm will move up and down while normal respiration occurs, but when it is stopped by a sharp edge of bone puncturing it, "shallow breathing" (short breaths) occurs. Also blood irritating the diaphragm will cause painful hiccuping. Unconsciousness, coma, and death are the usual results.

14

Striking the Spleen

Against a left cross, defender shuffles back into a cat stance as he catches the fist and locks the elbow of the attacker.

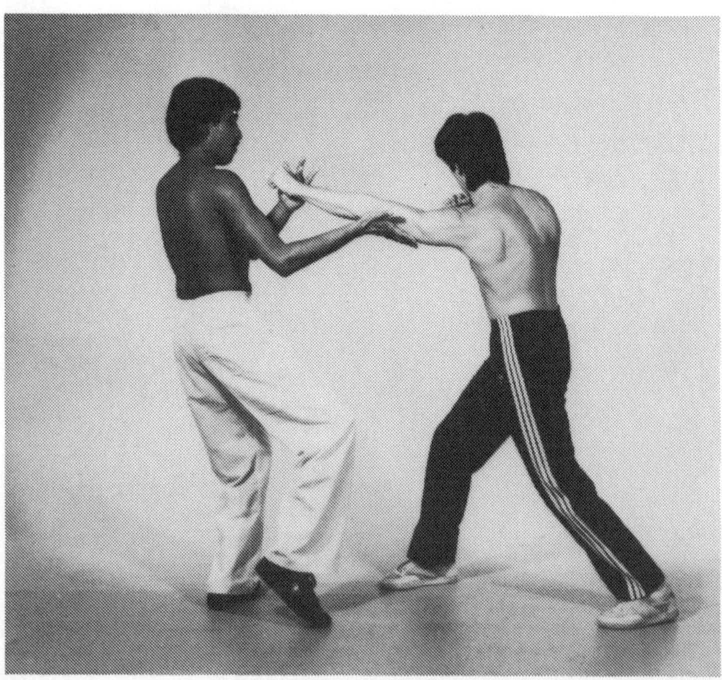

Defender pulls the attacker's arm through, pivots and delivers an instep kick to the attacker's spleen. This technique was completed in 6/10 of one second.

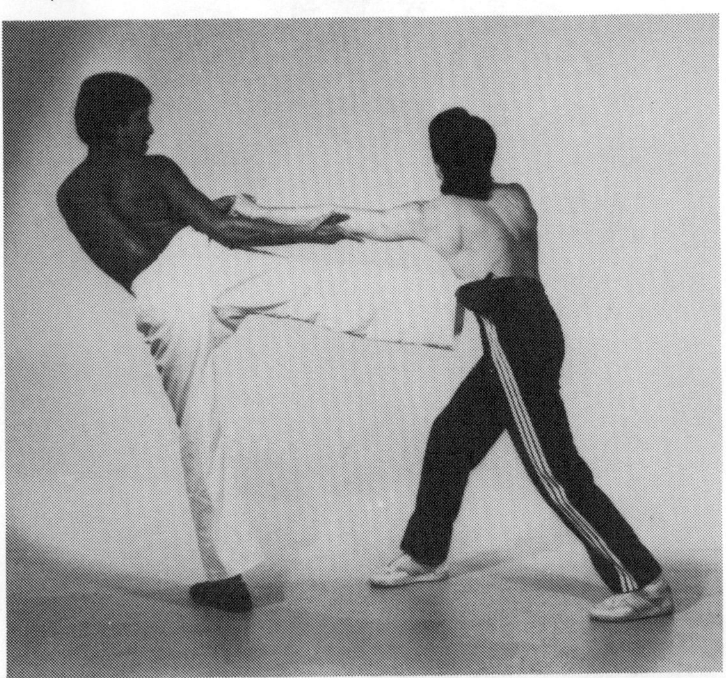

FIG. 47

TOP VIEW (NORMAL POSITIONS OF THE ORGANS IN THIS SECTON OF THE BODY)

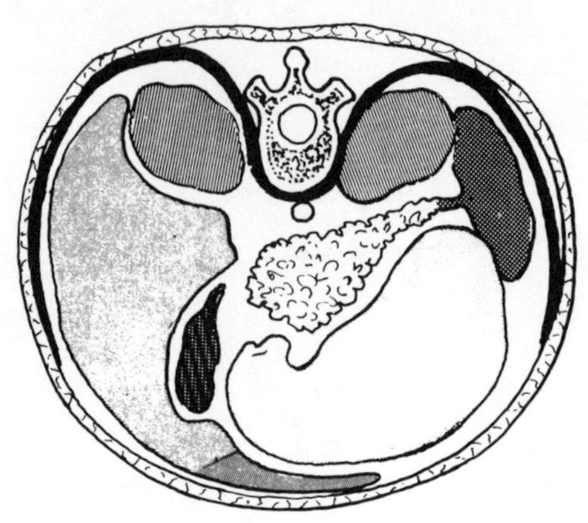

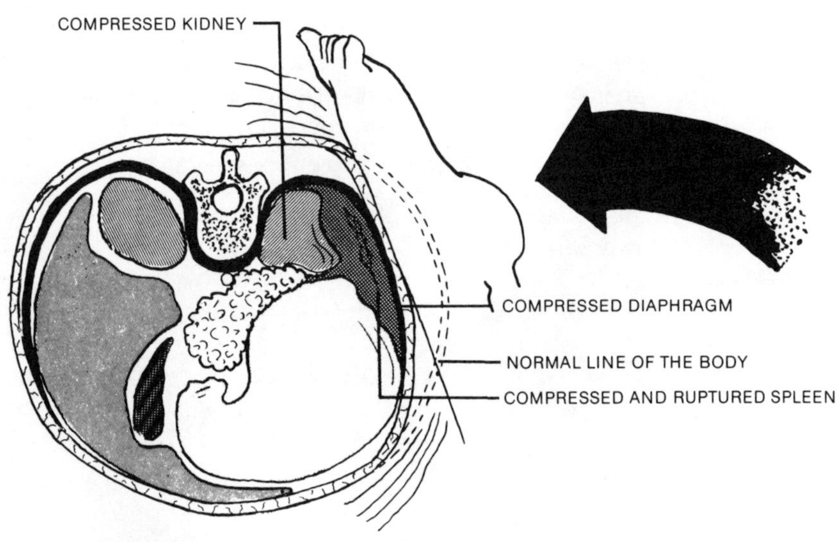

FIG. 48

NOTE: FLOATING RIBS LEFT OUT FOR CLARITY

WEAPON: Instep of the foot
TARGET: Spleen

Medical Implications

I. The spleen is located on the left side of the rib cage right beside the left kidney, under the diaphragm and parallel to the ninth, tenth and eleventh ribs. The function of the spleen that we are chiefly concerned with here is its ability to act as a reservoir for the storage of blood and to return it to normal circulation in harmony with the body's needs. During shock or fright, blood drains into the spleen and other internal organs. Under normal and stress situations the spleen is partially or nearly totally full of blood (according to the environment and emotions). (The spleen is also one of the main organs that fights against bodily infection, a very important function.)

II. A fracture of the ribs with lacerations of the diaphragm and spleen is the beginning of a slow but sure death.
Shock due to the loss of blood with weakness, nausea, severe pain and tenderness from the point of impact to the left side of the abdomen are the first symptoms; unconsciousness, coma, and death usually follow within forty-eight hours. Spasm of the diaphragm (Chapter 12) will also be present. Abdominal splinting is the hardening of the abdomen to a board-like ridgity due to the accumulation of a large amount of blood between the muscles and the abdominal cavity. Abdominal splinting will be a symptom in nearly all abdominal injuries. Pain in the abdomen and nausea occurs from the irritation of blood and bile in the abdominal cavity.

III. Even if the ribs are not fractured, a delayed rupture of the spleen may occur any time from within twenty-four hours to two years.* A small fissure or bruise, caused at the time of injury, can eventually increase in size and ultimately result in a massive hemorrhage with death the ultimate end. A delayed rupture of the spleen is almost always fatal because it is unexpected. A blow from the front or side can result in rupture of the spleen, especially if the opponent is inhaling when contact is made. During inhalation the muscles of the trunk are relaxed and very soft. This is evident by the easy pentration of a blow on inhalation.

* "Delayed rupture of the spleen" *Archives of Surgery* Vol. 92 No. 3, March 1966, p. 362.

15
Striking the Kidney

Against a left hook, defender steps to outside and positions left arm to parry attacker's punch.

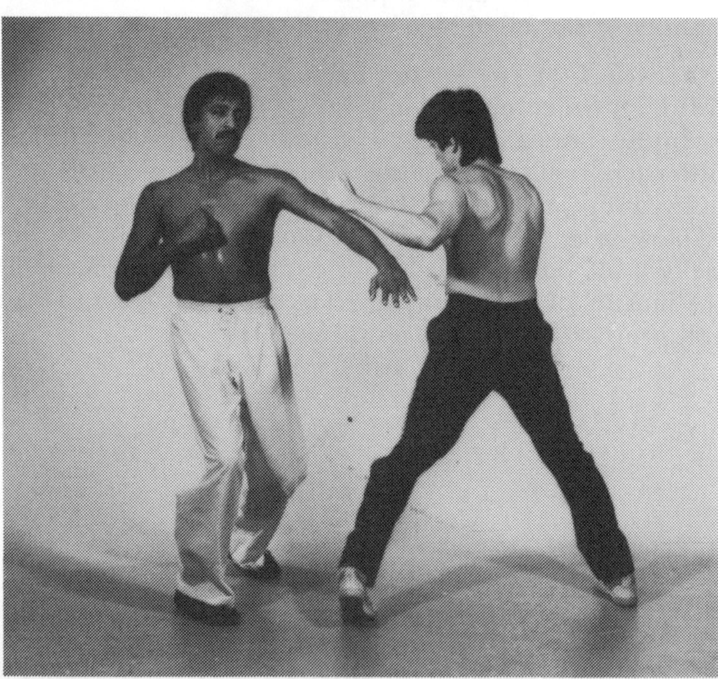

Defender drops to a low stance, parries the blow and cocks his right arm for an elbow strike.

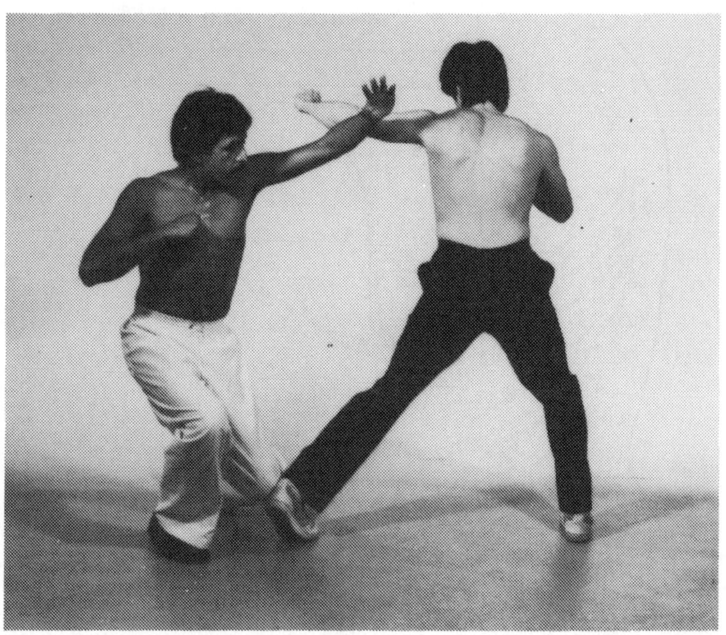

Defender pushes attacker around, pivots and strikes to the kidneys with his elbow. This technique was completed in 6/10 of one second.

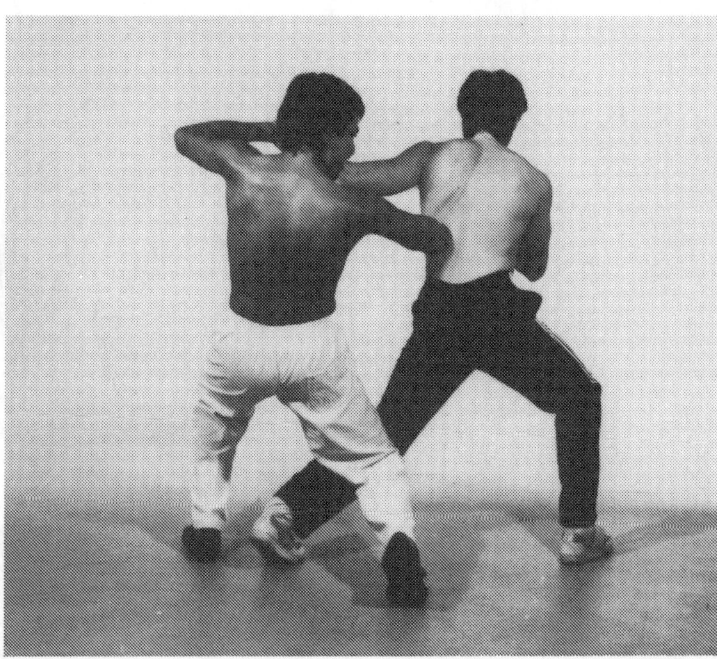

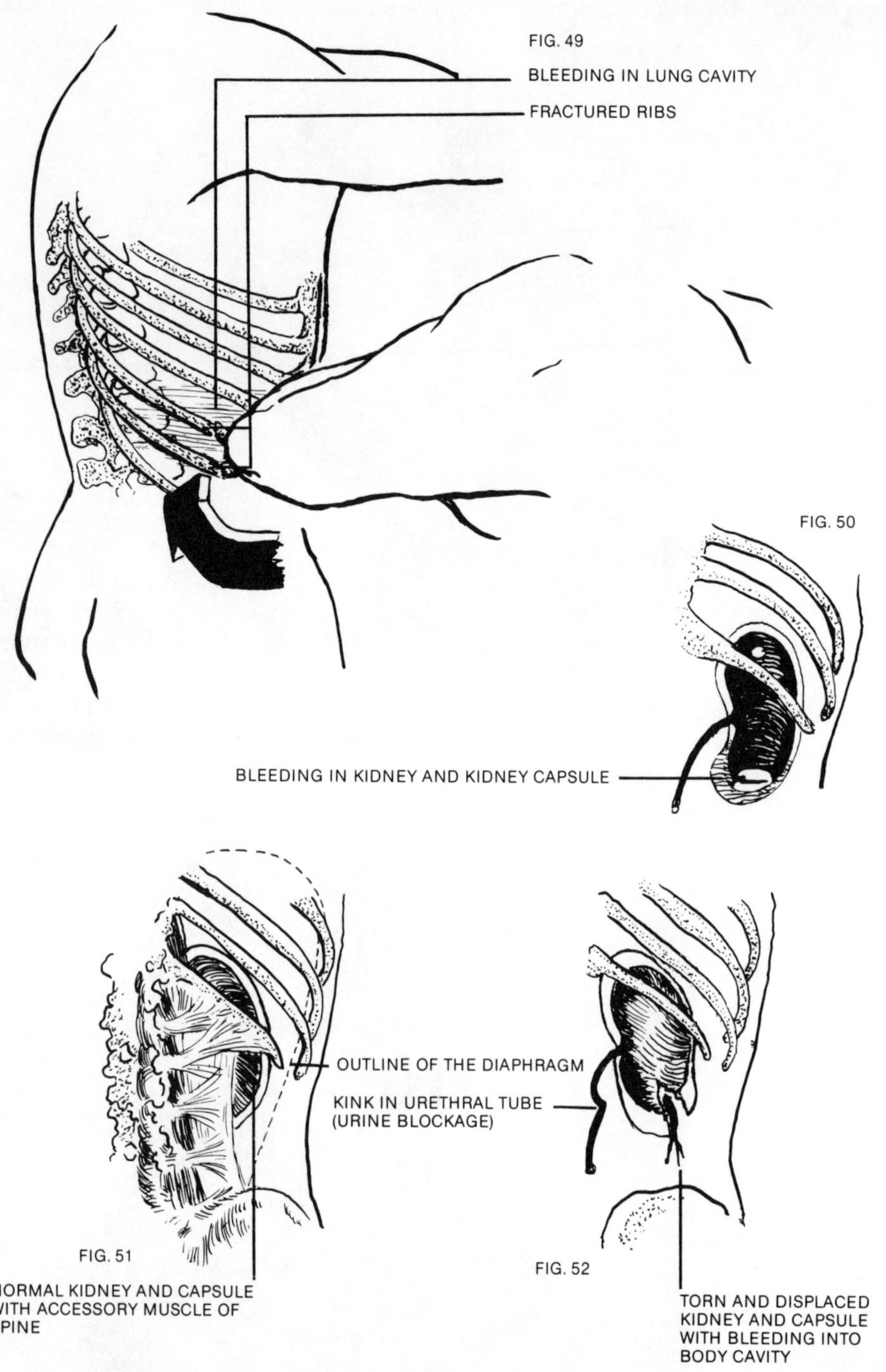

FIG. 49

FIG. 50

FIG. 51

FIG. 52

WEAPON: Elbow
TARGET: Kidney

Medical Implications

I. Rupture of the kidney, with bleeding in the capsule, can be prevalent with or without broken ribs. Hydrostatic pressure from the impact of the twelfth rib hitting the kidney can cause the rupture.

II. Laceration of the kidney from a broken rib is the most common type of injury from a blow of this nature. There will be peritonitis,* extreme pain, bloody urination, coma, and death (or at least many weeks in bed).

III. If the blow was a glancing type, just below the last rib (twelfth), the kidney capsule (membrane that holds kidney in place) would be torn from its moorings, causing bleeding into the body cavity; and because the ureter is displaced, a bend or kink in the ureter (urinary tube that goes to the bladder) would result in a urinary blockage, followed by infection and sometimes death.

IV. Because the diaphragm lies between the ribs and kidney, it will also be punctured if a complete break in the ribs has resulted. Spasms of the intercostal rib muscles and diaphragm will result in temporary to permanent respiratory paralysis with severe pain and ultimately death. (Chapter 12, Fig. 45.)

V. When the blow is three or four inches higher it may have an end result equal to that of a collapsed lung.

---

* Peritonitis is an accumulation of blood and urine irritating the abdominal walls—extreme tenderness of the abdomen.

16
Striking the Elbow

Against a lapel grab or palm push, defender pins the attackers wrist to his chest, steps back to pull and lock the elbow and cocks his left arm for a blow.

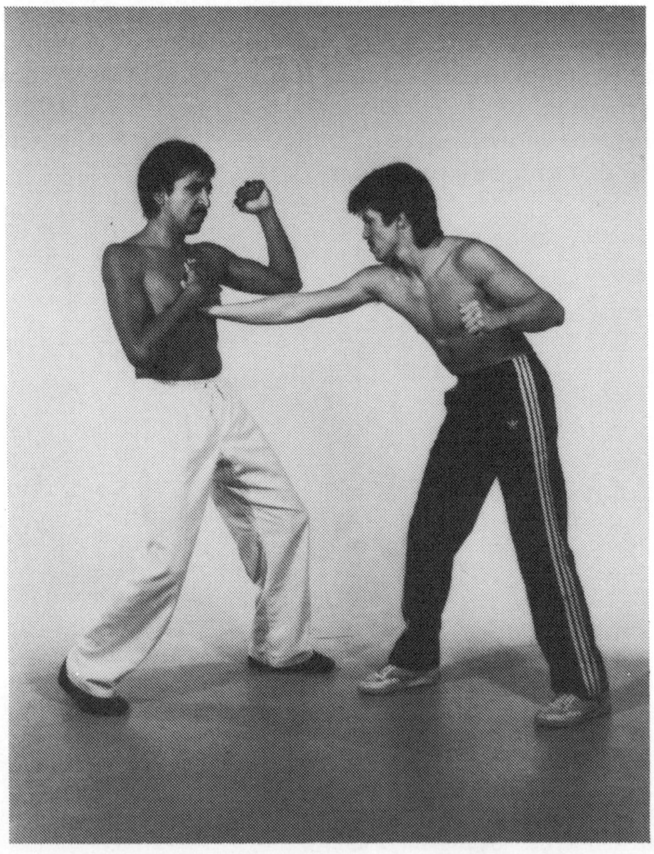

Defender pivots, twisting the attacker's arm and strikes with his elbow just above the locked joint, hyperextending the elbow and/or shoulder. This technique was completed in 7/10 of one second.

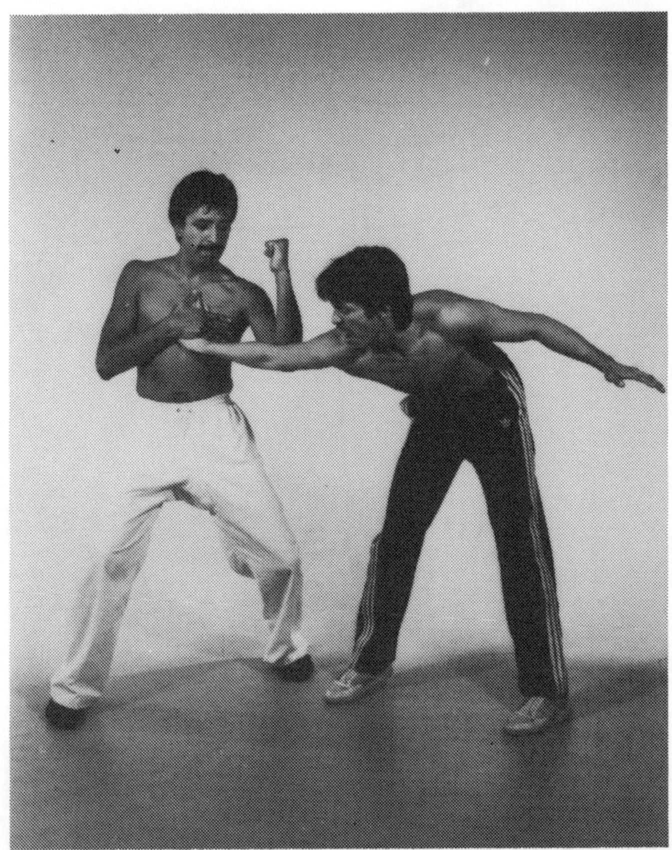

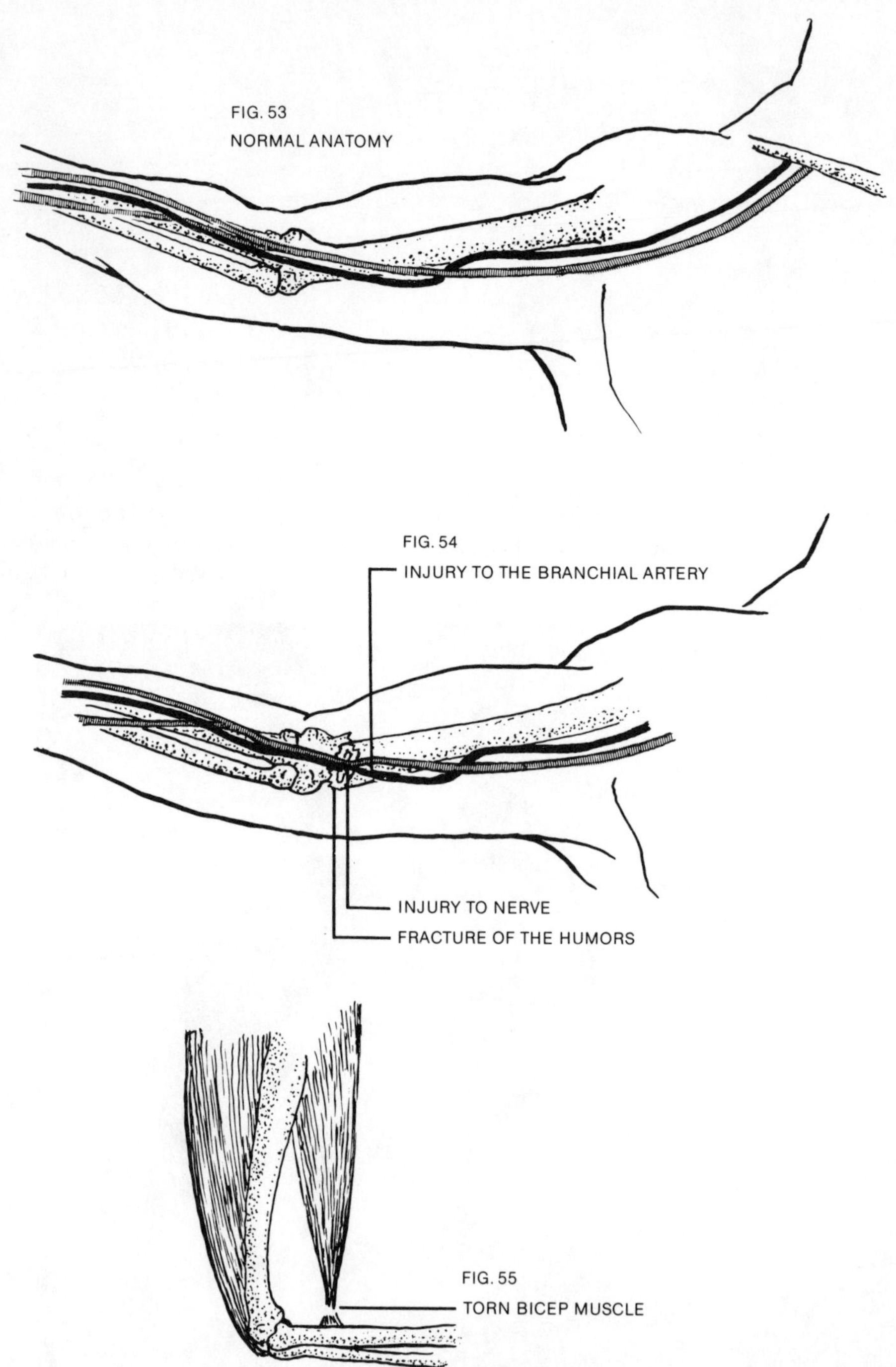

FIG. 53
NORMAL ANATOMY

FIG. 54

FIG. 55

WEAPON: Forearm
TARGET: Elbow

Medical Implications

I. Fracture of the humorus will result when the blow is slightly above the elbow joint. In injuries to the upper arm, the ulna and sometimes the radial and median nerves may be pinched or severed by the broken bone, resulting in slight to permanent paralysis of parts of the arm and/or hand. Nausea, anxiety, and extreme pain accompany this trauma.
II. Injury to the branchial artery in an unwelcome complication of the fracture because a pinched or severed blood vessel may result in tissue damage or gangrene. Four to six hours is all that is needed to produce this condition. Loss of sensation and amputation of the arm is the irreversible outcome.

III. "Tennis elbow" can be a very devastating injury. A torn bursa (lubricating sac of the elbow joint) will cause a swelling of tremendous size in and around the elbow. Extreme pain in the elbow when extension of the arm is attempted is the adhering symptom. Joint motion may be limited because of adhesions within the muscles (biceps, etc.) and tendons surrounding the joint.

17

Striking the Bladder

Against a right cross, defender sidesteps and blocks the punch with his left forearm, readying his right arm and fist for a counterstrike.

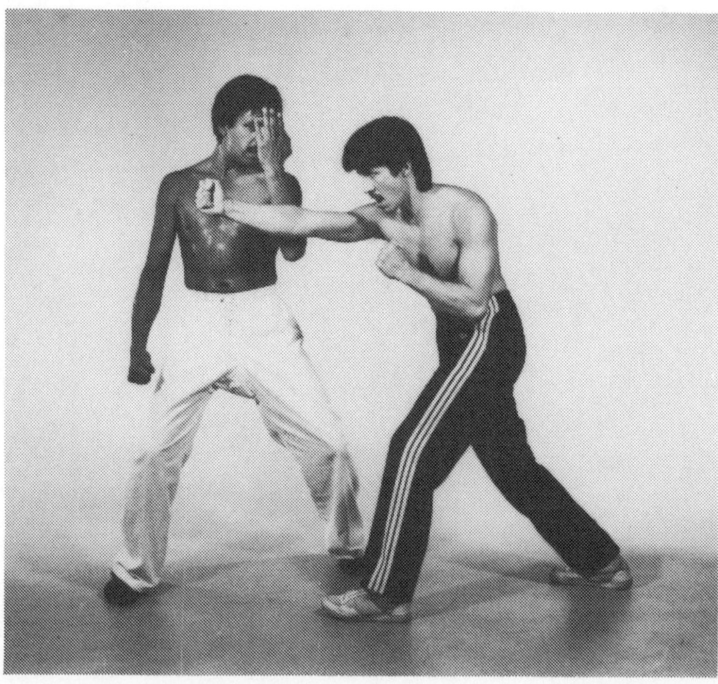

Defender swings the attacker's arm down and out as he pivots to add power to the upward blow.

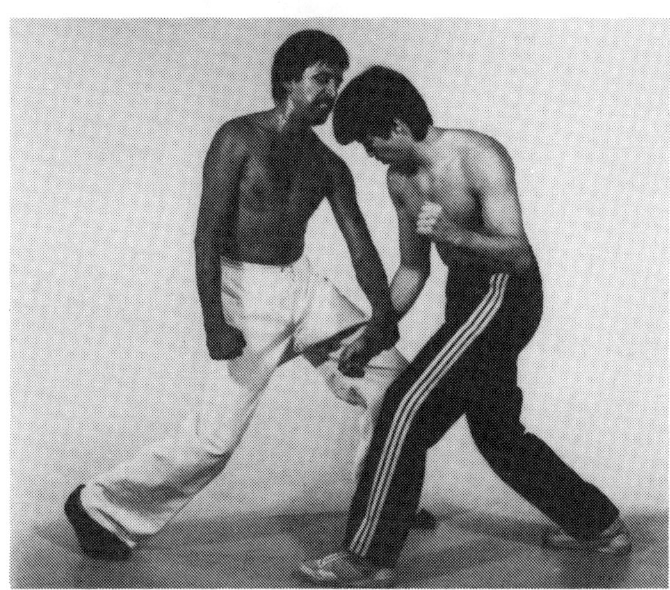

Defender strikes to attacker's bladder with a reverse hammerfist. This technique was completed in 7/10 of one second.

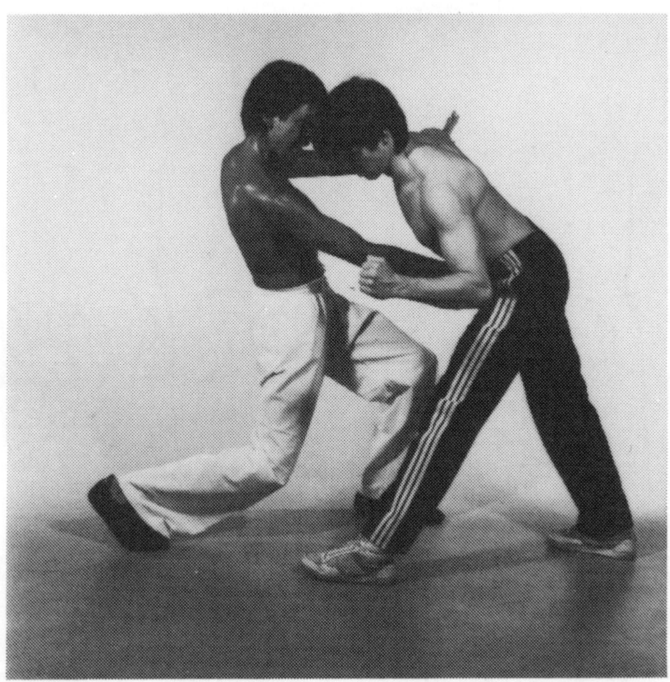

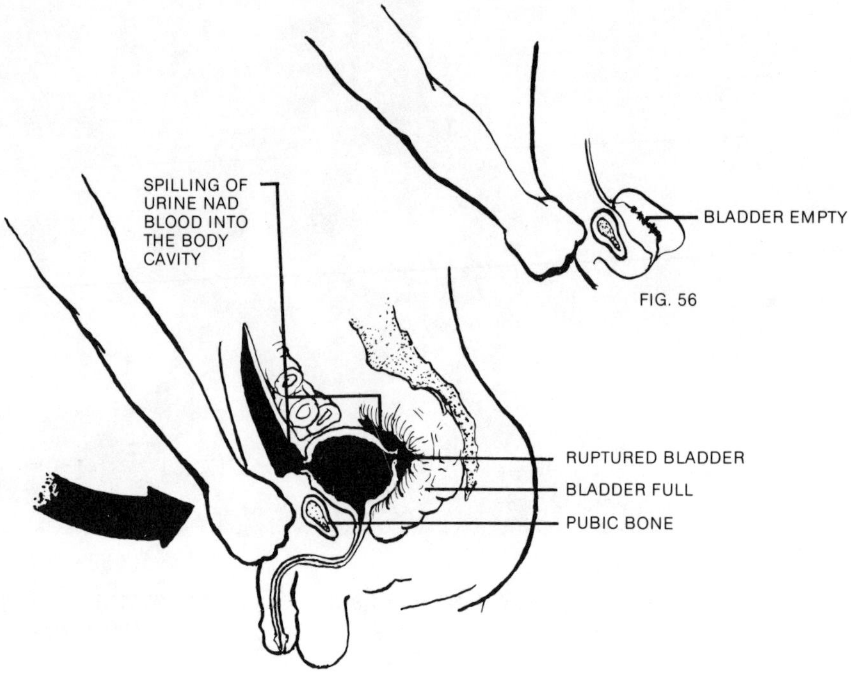

FIG. 56

FIG. 57

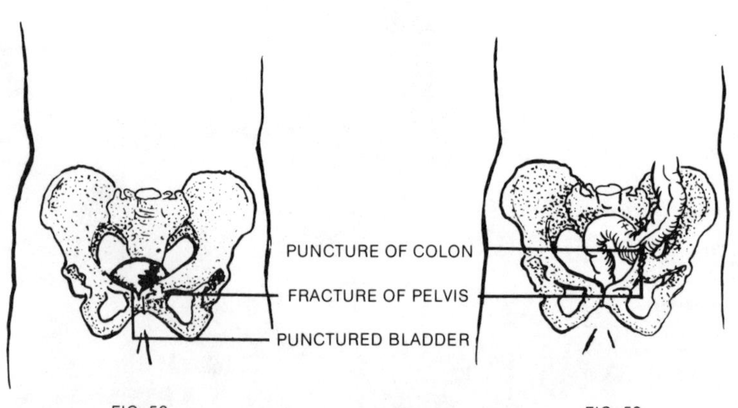

FIG. 58

FIG. 59

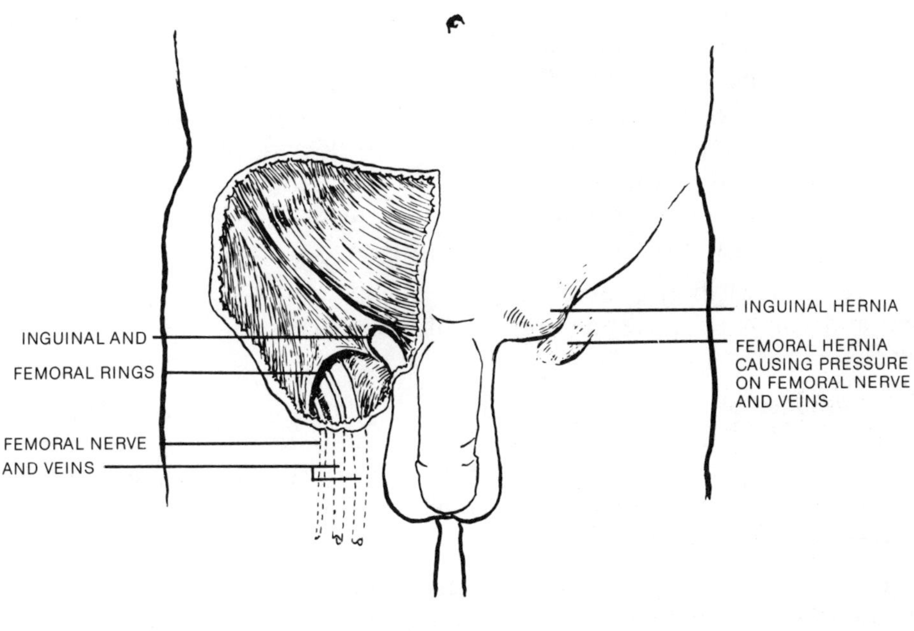

FIG. 60

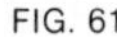
FIG. 61

THROMBOSIS (BLOOD CLOT IN THE VESSEL, CLOGGING NORMAL CIRCULATION)

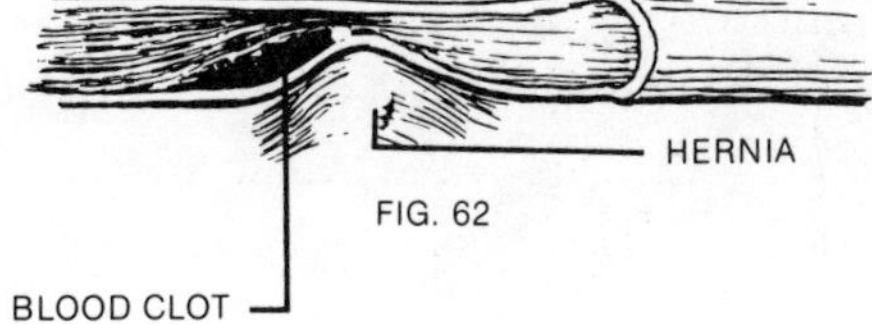

FIG. 62

WEAPON: Reverse Hammerfist
TARGET: Bladder

Medical Implications

I. Rupture of the urinary bladder in its distended (full) state is equivalent to filling a balloon with air until a weak portion of the balloon ruptures and releases its contents, which in this case is urine. The area of the bladder will have a strained feeling with increasing tenderness from spilled urine and blood in the body cavity. Inability to urinate more than a few bloody drops of urine—if at all—is an indication of a rupture of the bladder or urethral passageway (tube leading from the bladder to the outside). Infection due to lesions in the tube or bladder cause urinary retention, muscle spasm of the bladder, or painful and frequent urination. Infection seems to be an accomplice of nearly all urinary injuries.

II. A really hard driving blow (slightly lower) would fracture the pubic bone and consequently puncture the bladder (with the same results as above).

III. A fracture of the top edge of the pubic bone may easily produce a punctured colon (intestine) if an off-center blow to the left side of the opponent occurs. Respiration will be difficult because of the pressure downward of the intestinal tract upon the fractured bone segment. Hemorrhage and shock conclude this injury.

IV. Because of the wide area of this blow and the narrowing delta-like region of the lower abdomen, a possible inguinal or femoral hernia may develop if the blow is a few inches lower on either side of the bladder. This occurs basically because of the already weakened and thin inguinal and femoral muscle rings. The inguinal and femoral rings are the byproduct of a number of muscles disecting at various angles to produce a whirlpool effect with a hole in the center.
In the inguinal ring, the spermatic cord (cord leading to the testicle) emerges from this hole. When the surrounding muscle is weakened from a tear or disruption of the muscle fibers, portions of the bowl, bladder, and/or omentum (abdominal membrane) may protrude through the weakened muscle ring and continue into the scrotum (scrotal hernia). This is the usual discomforting after-effect of a strong blow in this region.

V. Two related complications may become prevalent in a femoral hernia. The femoral and iliac vein and the femoral nerve run through or by the ring orifice.

a.) Protruding parts of the bowl, or omentum, may become constricted from pressure of the expanded ring around them. These parts may become gangrenous from lack of blood. Of course, pressure on the femorial nerve if severe enough will cause partial paralysis of the lower limb.

b.) Thrombosis* in the femorial vein (depending upon how great the thrombosis) can ultimately lodge in the lungs and cause death.

* Thrombosis: Blood clot in the vessel, clogging circulation.

18
Striking the Groin

Defender is caught in a two-hand front choke, attacker's thumbs are pressing into the throat.

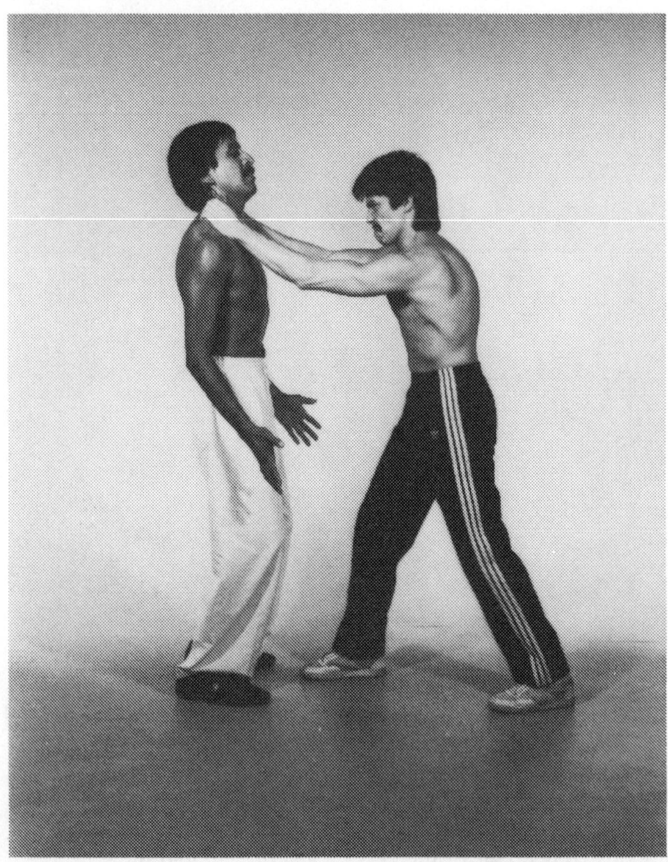

Defender steps back and drops into a cat stance as he slaps the attacker's arms together and pushes them up.

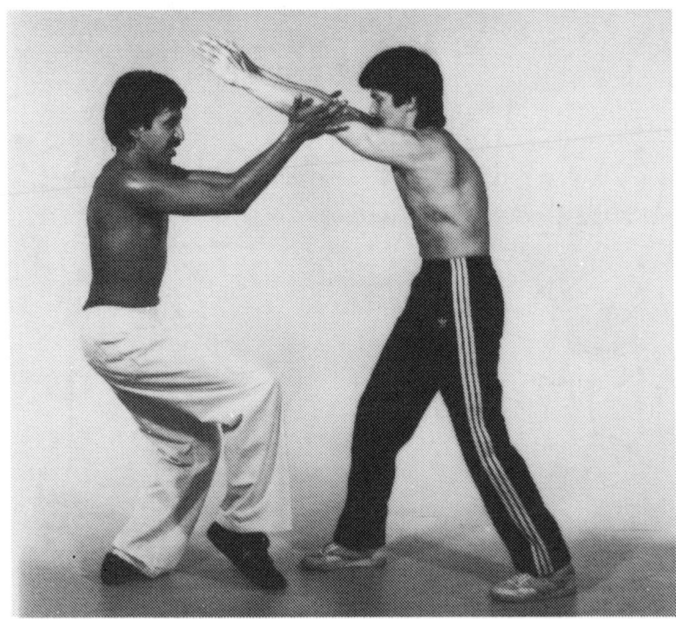

Defender kicks to the groin. This technique was completed in 7/10 of one second.

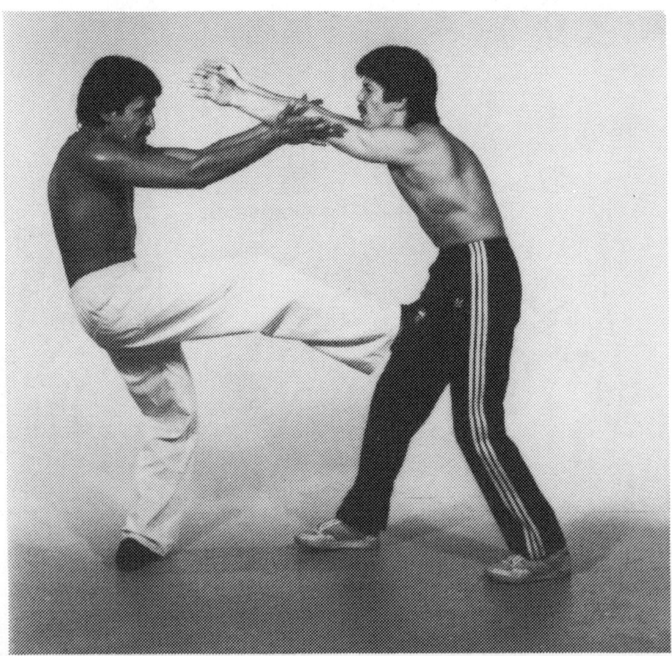

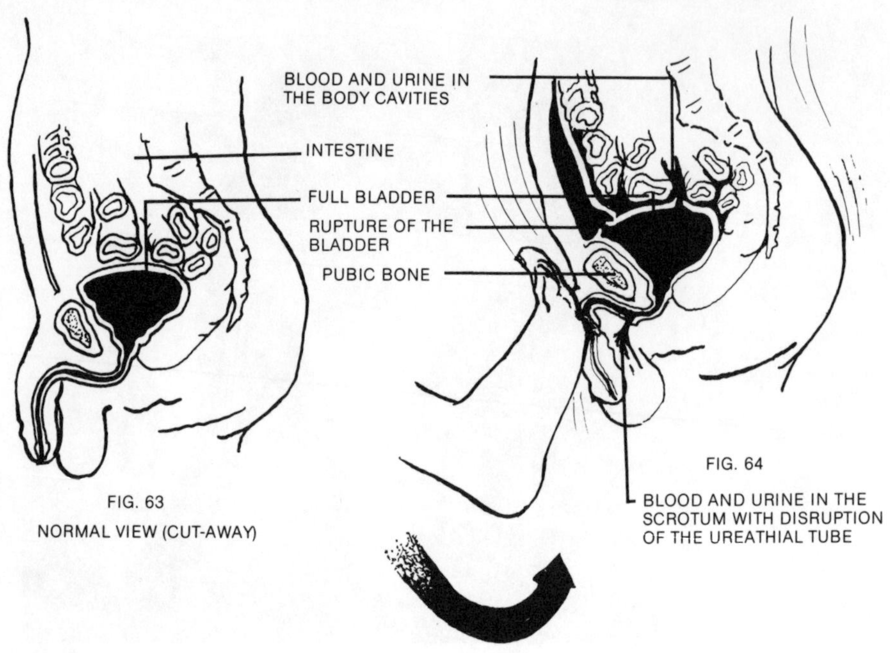

FIG. 63
NORMAL VIEW (CUT-AWAY)

FIG. 64

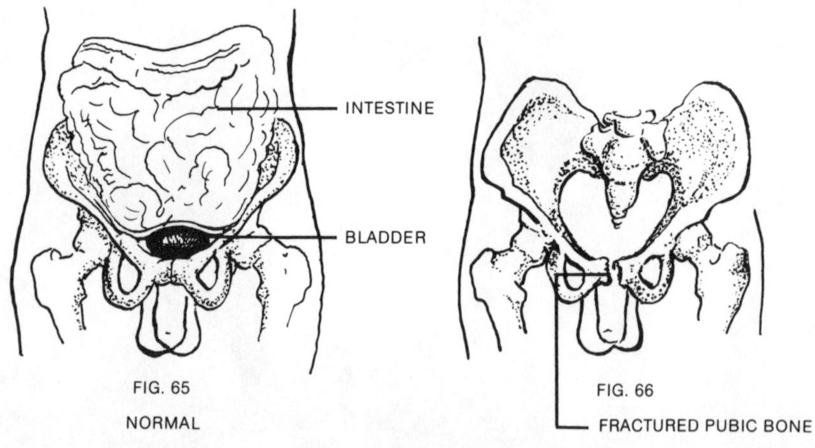

FIG. 65
NORMAL

FIG. 66

WEAPON: Ball of foot
TARGET: Groin

Medical Implications

I. Rupture of the bladder from the percussive jolt of a solid kick or from a fracture of the pubic bone, are the two main methods of rupture (other than the method already mentioned in the previous chapter). Blood and urine in the abdominal cavity will be in abundance with the usual tenderness and pain.

II. The center of the pubic bone is the weakest and most probable place of fracture. An inability to walk because of the nauseating pain originating between the legs (due to the pinching, abrading effect of the separated pubic bones rubbing together upon attempted movement) will leave your opponent in a distressed prone position.

III. In order for the kick to penetrate to the underside of the frontal pubic bone, it must first drive through the penis and scrotum (not a very difficult feat). Disruption of the urethra (urinary tube leading to the outside) with bleeding and urine into the scrotum will be the minimal injury. Bloody and painful urination or an inability to urinate will more than likely be the aftermath.

IV. The testicles are extremely mobile within the loose skin of the scrotum; however, a crushed testicle may result, due to the wide surface of the ball of the foot striking it. Sterility to one or both testicles is one sure occurrence from such a heavy blow. Pain, shock, loss of breath, nausea, vomiting, unconsciousness (and sometimes death) commonly follow one another.

19

Striking the Spine

Against a tackle, defender steps back, cocks his left arm and catches attacker's head with his right hand.

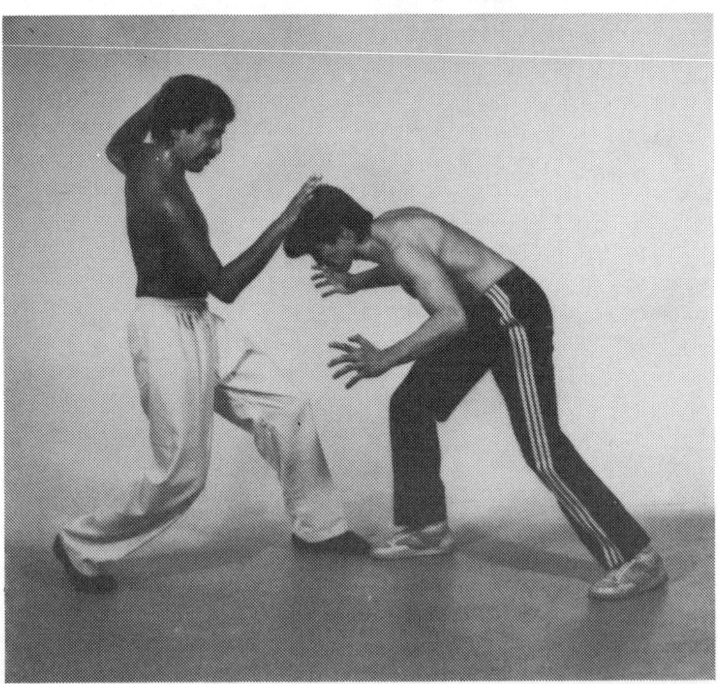

Defender's right hand directs attacker's head down and forward. Defender pivots and strikes with the elbow to the spine. This technique was completed in 4/10 of one second.

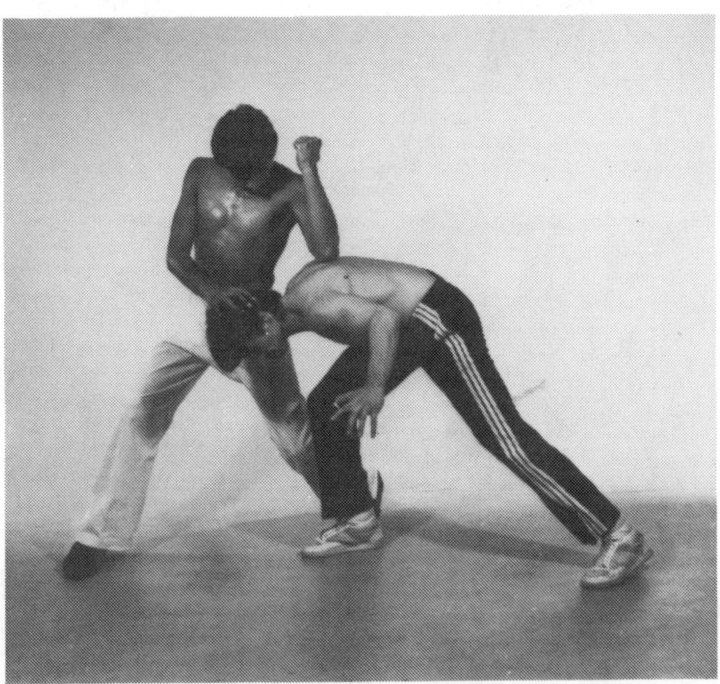

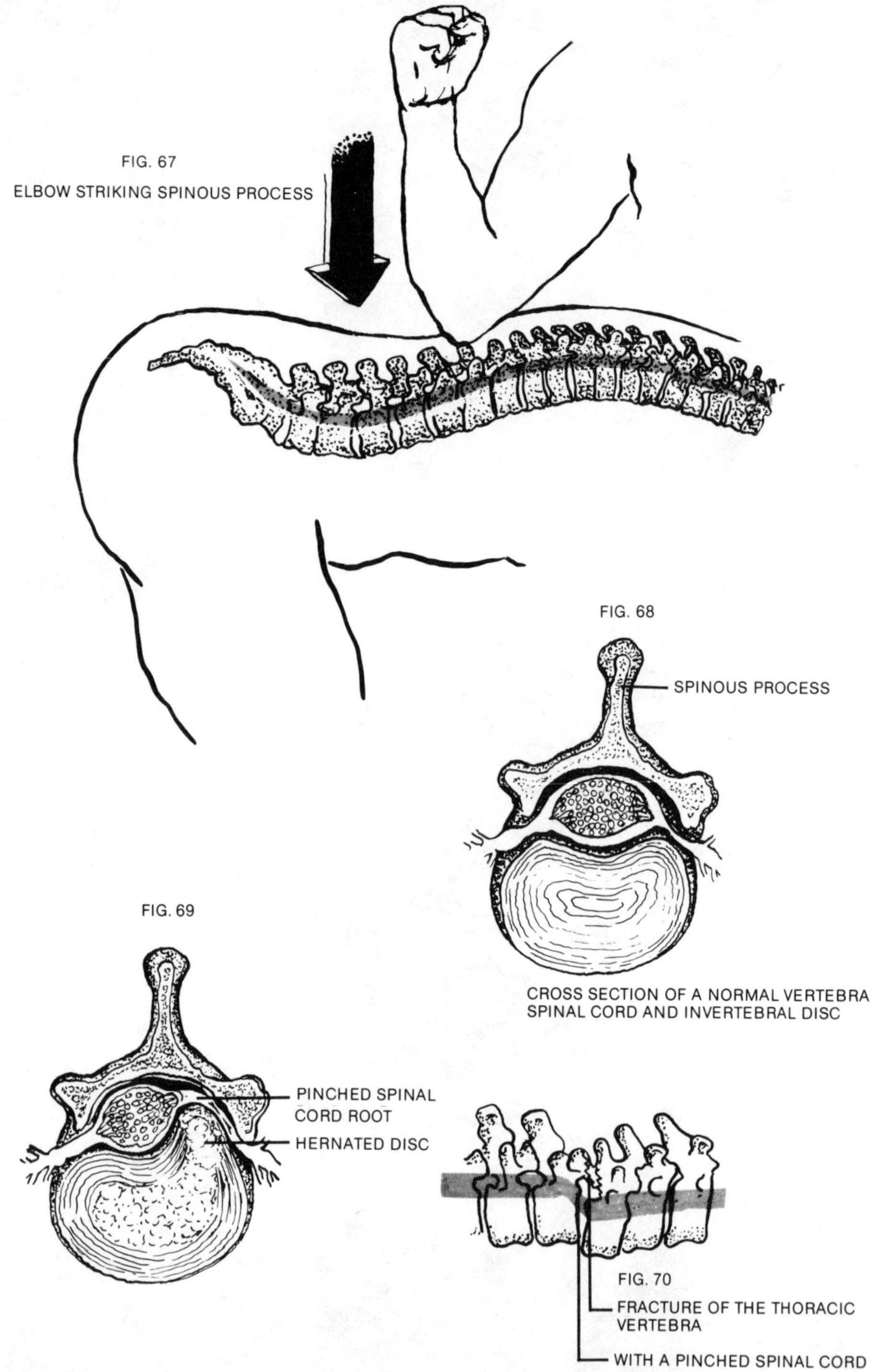

FIG. 67
ELBOW STRIKING SPINOUS PROCESS

FIG. 68
CROSS SECTION OF A NORMAL VERTEBRA
SPINAL CORD AND INVERTEBRAL DISC

FIG. 69

FIG. 70

WEAPON: Elbow
TARGET: Spine

Medical Implications

I. A fracture of the thoracic vertebra and intervertebral disc will quickly neutralize your opponent. Paralysis of the body below the point of impact will predominate if the crushed vertebra or disc has severed or created enough direct pressure to compress the spinal cord. Loss of control of the bladder and rectum from paralysis is a distressing adjustment. The higher up on the spine the blow was struck, the more areas involved in paralysis. Quite often urinary infection results because of the paralyzed bladder.

II. Pressure in the spinal cord due to a hemorrhage there may produce partial to complete paralysis (without the presence of a crushed vertebra or disc exerting pressure upon the cord).

III. Minor results, if you have withheld the force of the blow, will be a pinched nerve root (nerve strand leaving the vertebra and connecting to any number of muscle or organ groups throughout the body) causing slight paralysis and malfunction of certain areas. This is often termed a slipped disc or herniated disc (Figure 69). Extrusion of the disc (herniated disc) into the region of the cord may terminate in partial to complete motor and/or sensory loss or uncontrollable spastic movement. This may be a later effect.

IV. Spinal cord shock ("whiplash"), without visible disruption of the cord fibers, will radiate violent pain up and down the spinal cord.

V. If the blow slipped off or missed the vertebra by a fraction of an inch and struck hard, it would easily collapse the lung (Chapter 12) from the percussive shock of the blow or from a fractured rib.

20

Striking the Thigh

Against a roundkick, defender steps back and to the inside of attacker's kick, preparing to block the kick with his left arm.

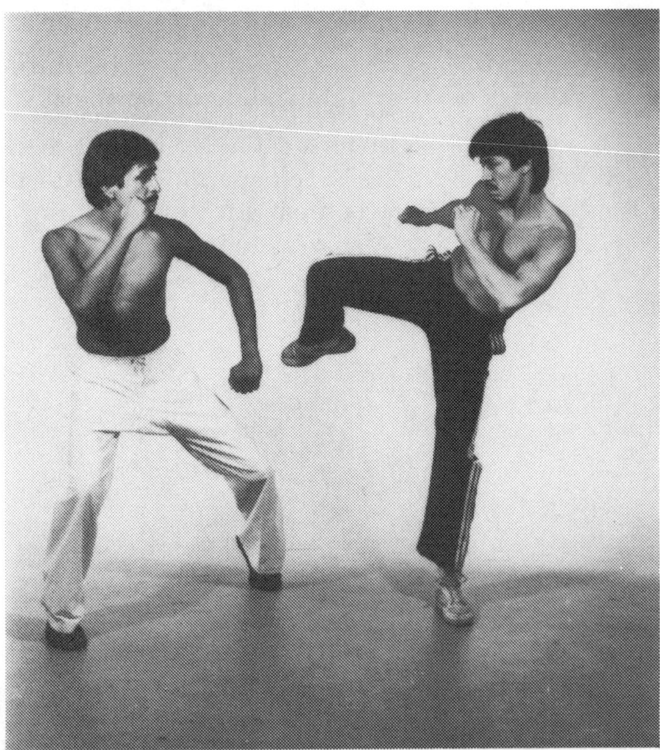

Defender hooks attacker's leg, pulls it straight and prepares to strike with his right knee and elbow.

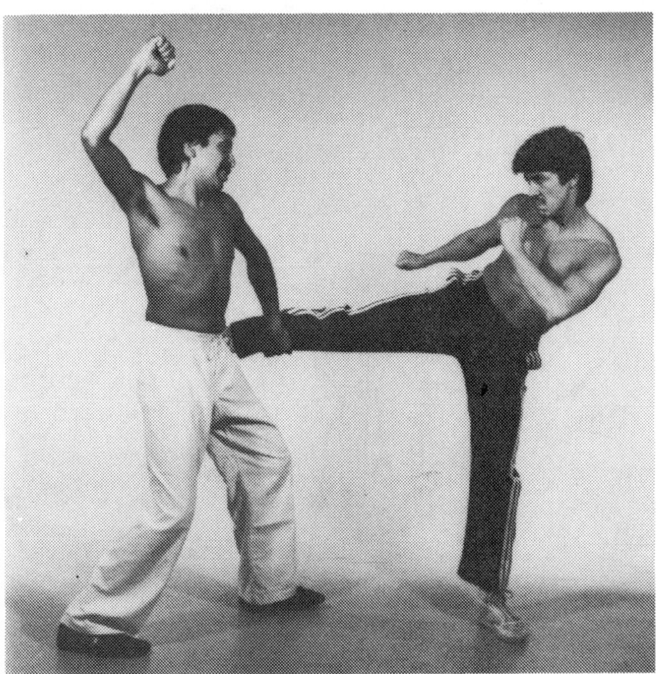

Defender simultaneously strikes to the underside of thigh with his knee and to the top of the thigh with his elbow. This technique was completed in 8/10 of one second.

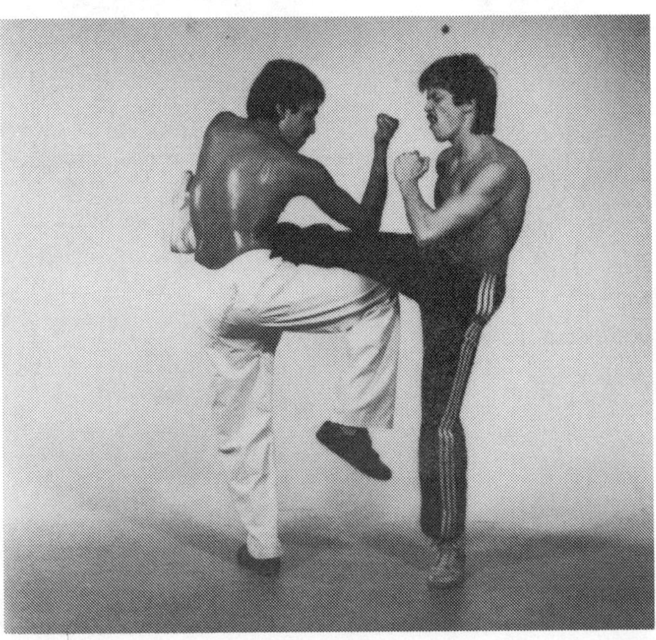

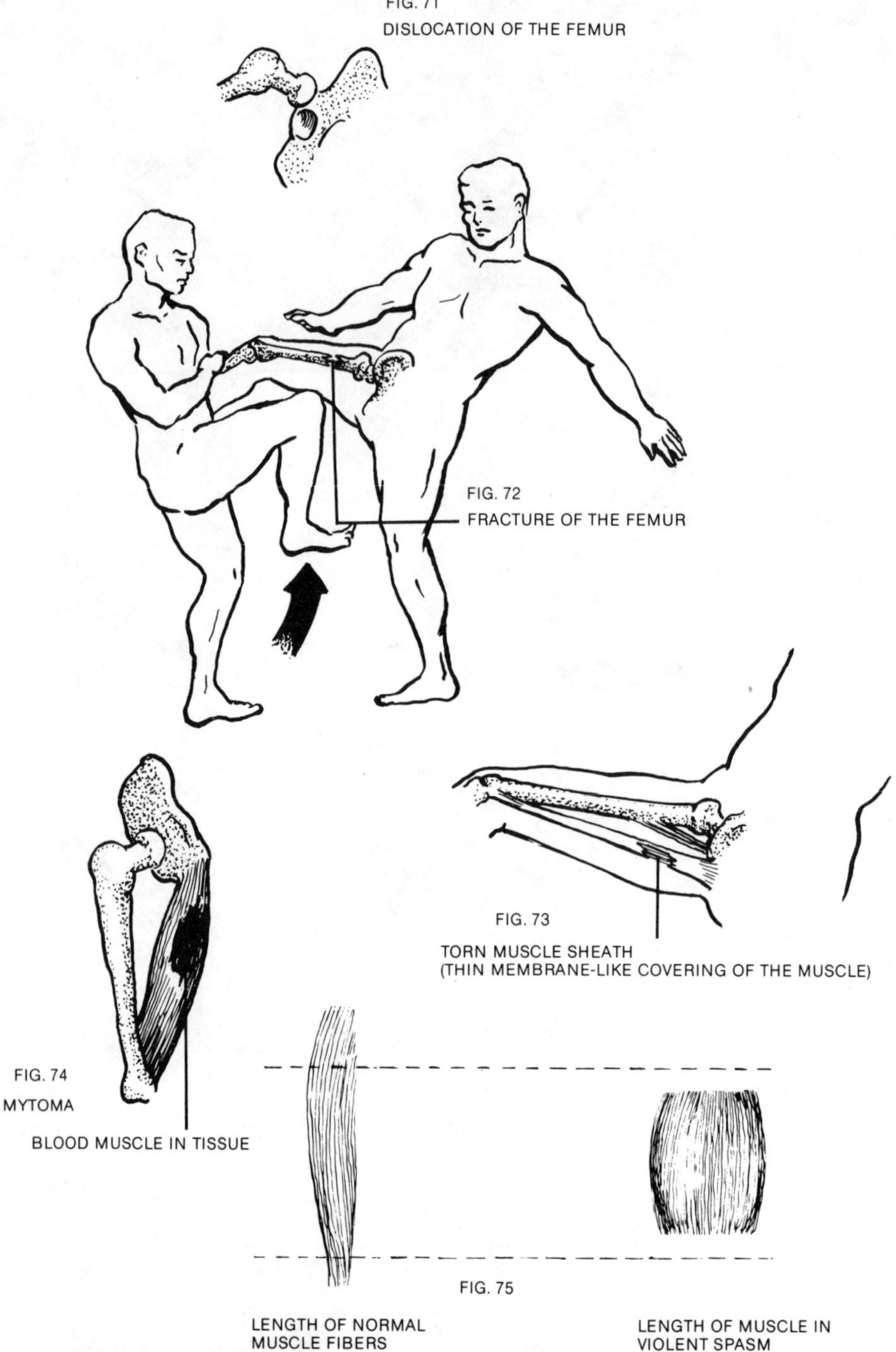
FIG. 71
DISLOCATION OF THE FEMUR
FIG. 72
FRACTURE OF THE FEMUR
FIG. 73
TORN MUSCLE SHEATH
(THIN MEMBRANE-LIKE COVERING OF THE MUSCLE)
FIG. 74
MYTOMA
BLOOD MUSCLE IN TISSUE
FIG. 75
LENGTH OF NORMAL
MUSCLE FIBERS
LENGTH OF MUSCLE IN
VIOLENT SPASM

WEAPON: Knee
TARGET: Underside of the thigh

Medical Implications

I. This technique is one that should be used only when the attacker has demonstrated an inadequate attempt to deliver a slow or sloppy kick. Ultimately, this blow (one of the strongest human weapons) will fracture or dislocate the femur. The result is severe: many months in a fracture bed with immediate immobility and possible shock because of the harsh pain. Severe muscle spasm (Figure 75) will be prevalent with any hard blow to a muscle.

II. Disruption of the muscle sheath and bleeding in the muscle fibre (mytoma) are the common outcome. Herniation of the muscle tissues is a result of the torn muscle sheath (thin membrane covering) that normally covers and binds the muscle groups and fibers together. Without the restricting pressure of the membrane around the muscle, a protrusion of the injured muscle fibre through the torn membrane will create a lump on the point of impact. Many months of immobility due to loss of contracting ability of the muscle are sure to follow.

21

Striking the Back of the Knee

Against an overhead club strike, defender steps to the outside and redirects the blow downward.

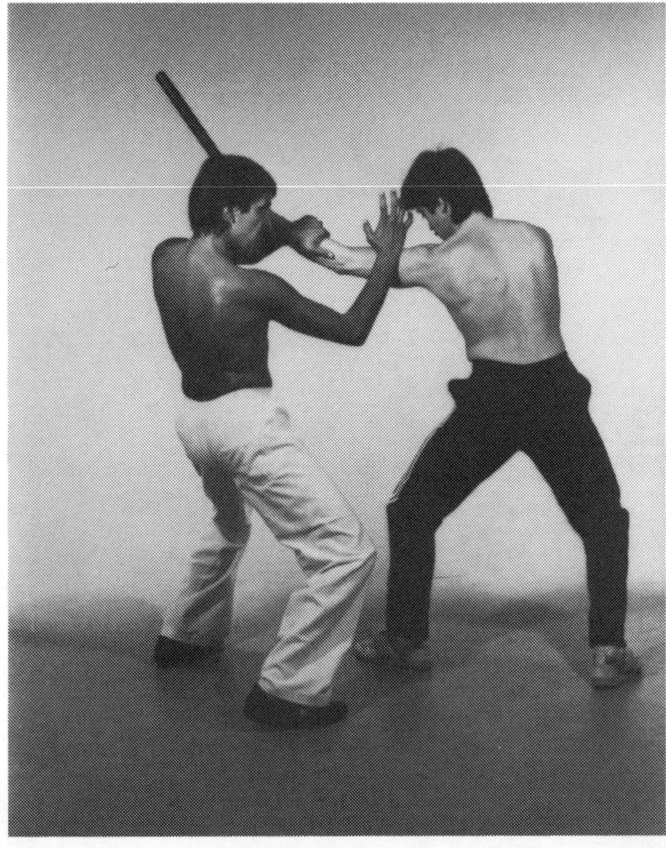

Defender steps through and prepares to deliver a downward heelkick, simultaneously pulling the attacker's arm with his left hand, and the attacker's shoulder with his right hand.

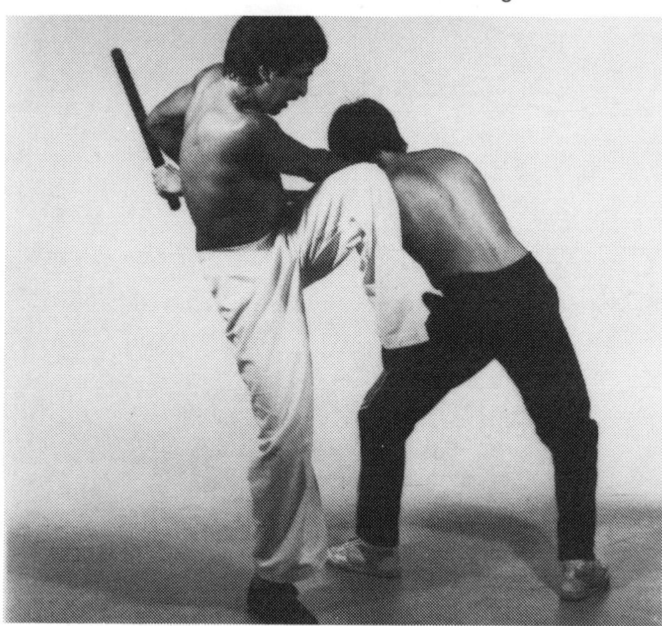

Defender delivers the heelkick to the back of the attacker's right knee while twisting his torso to pull the attacker toward him. This technique was completed in 8/10 of one second.

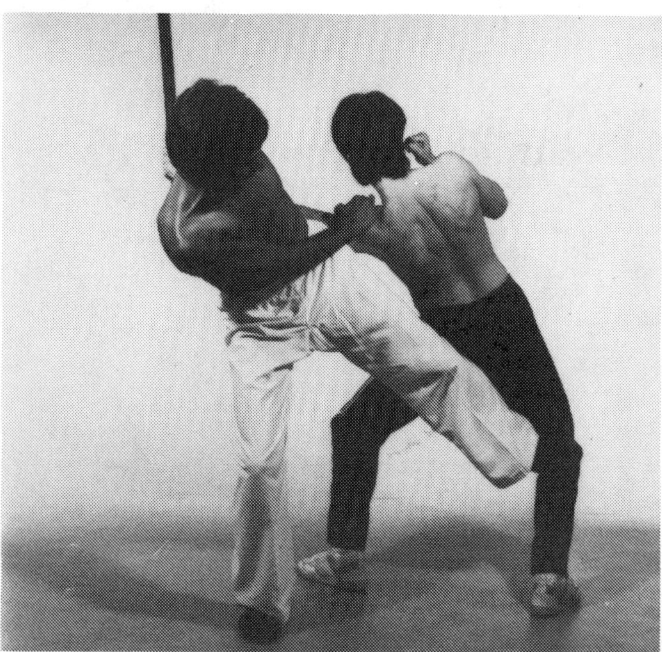

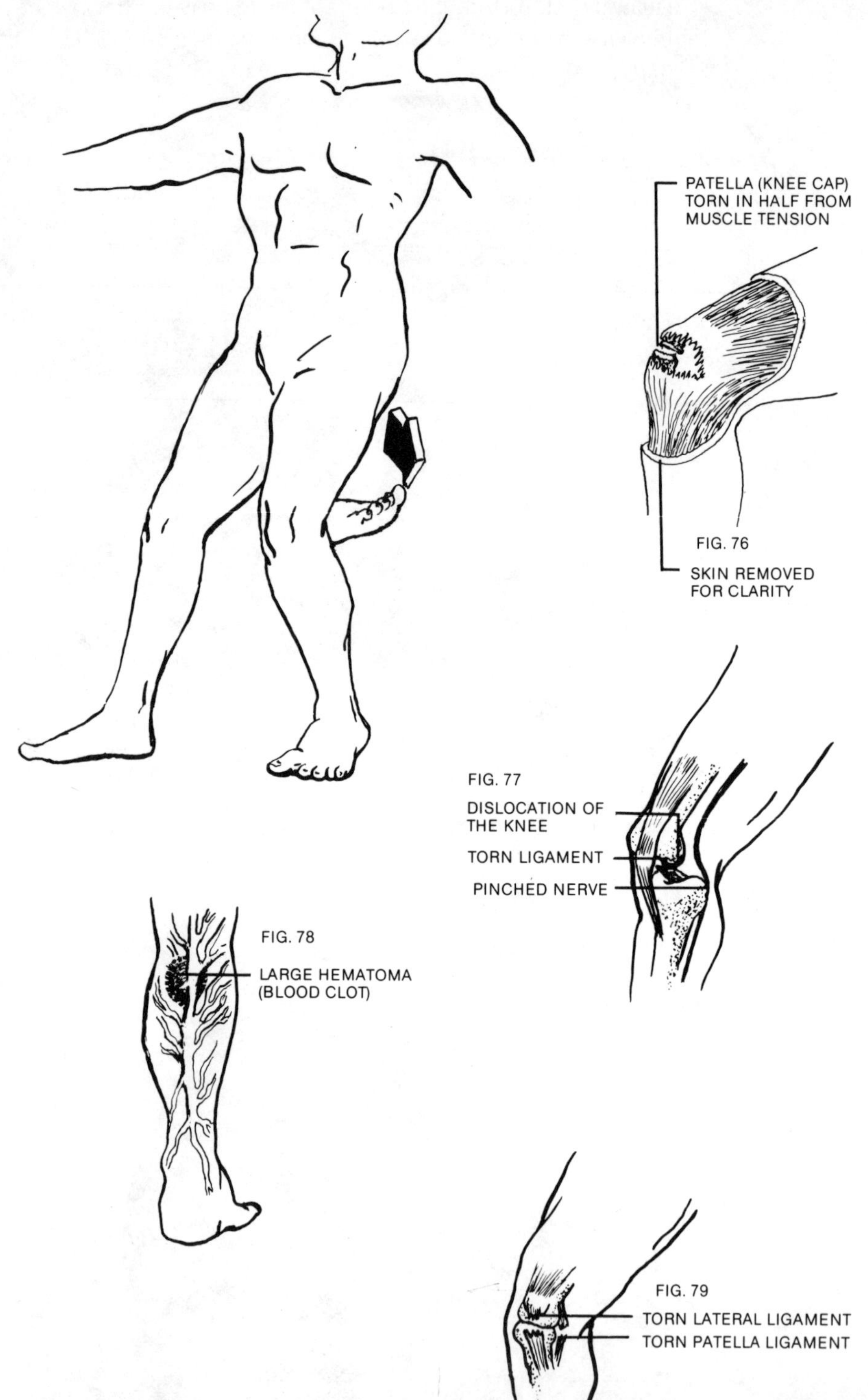
PATELLA (KNEE CAP)
TORN IN HALF FROM
MUSCLE TENSION
FIG. 76
SKIN REMOVED
FOR CLARITY
FIG. 77
DISLOCATION OF
THE KNEE
TORN LIGAMENT
PINCHED NERVE
FIG. 78
LARGE HEMATOMA
(BLOOD CLOT)
FIG. 79
TORN LATERAL LIGAMENT
TORN PATELLA LIGAMENT

WEAPON: Knife edge of foot
TARGET: Back of knee

Medical Implications

I. The popliteal blood vessels and tabialis nerve run together up and down the backside of the leg, so when one is affected the other usually is also. A torn blood vessel and abrasion of the nerve can easily result from a kick of this nature (especially when a shoe is worn). A large hematoma (an organized area of blood spilled from a torn blood vessel) will form under the skin and sometimes the swelling will extend forward to the front of the knee. An abrasion of the nerve will cause partial paralysis of the leg below the point of impact; the mobility of the knee will be greatly impaired to say the least.

II. When the knee is thrust forward and the upper body is jerked back, the muscle tension on the knee is so great that it can tear all of the muscles of the knee; often the muscle action has torn the kneecap in half. Repair of such violent trauma is major in effect and must be done soon or the muscles will not grow back in the proper places. The great pain and torn muscles will render your opponent virtually helpless.

III. If a dislocation of the knee joint has occurred, it would undoubtedly be the most painful result that could happen to the knee. Surgical repositioning of the ripped muscles and ligaments are a necessary course of action if that individual ever wishes to walk again. Shock, nausea, and pain are the immediate effect.

22 Striking the Front Knee Joint

Against a right handed knife thrust, the defender parries the thrust across his body as he steps back into a cat stance.

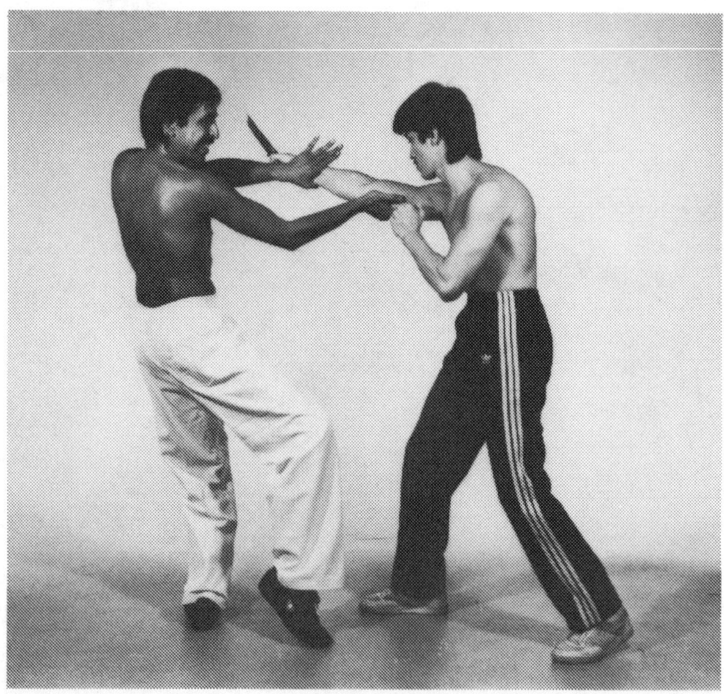

Defender pulls the attacker's arm straight as he cocks his leg for the kick.

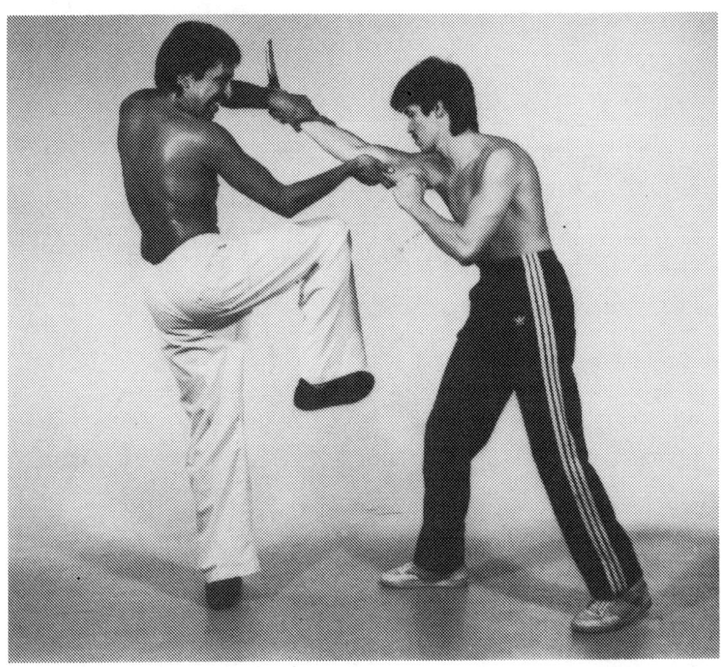

Defender pivots and strikes with the side of his foot to the opponent's knee. This technique was completed in 7/10 of one second.

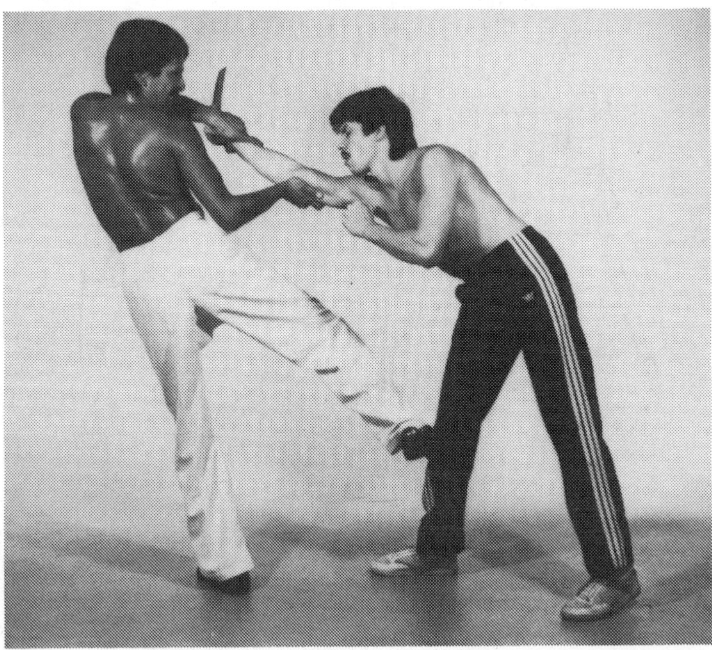

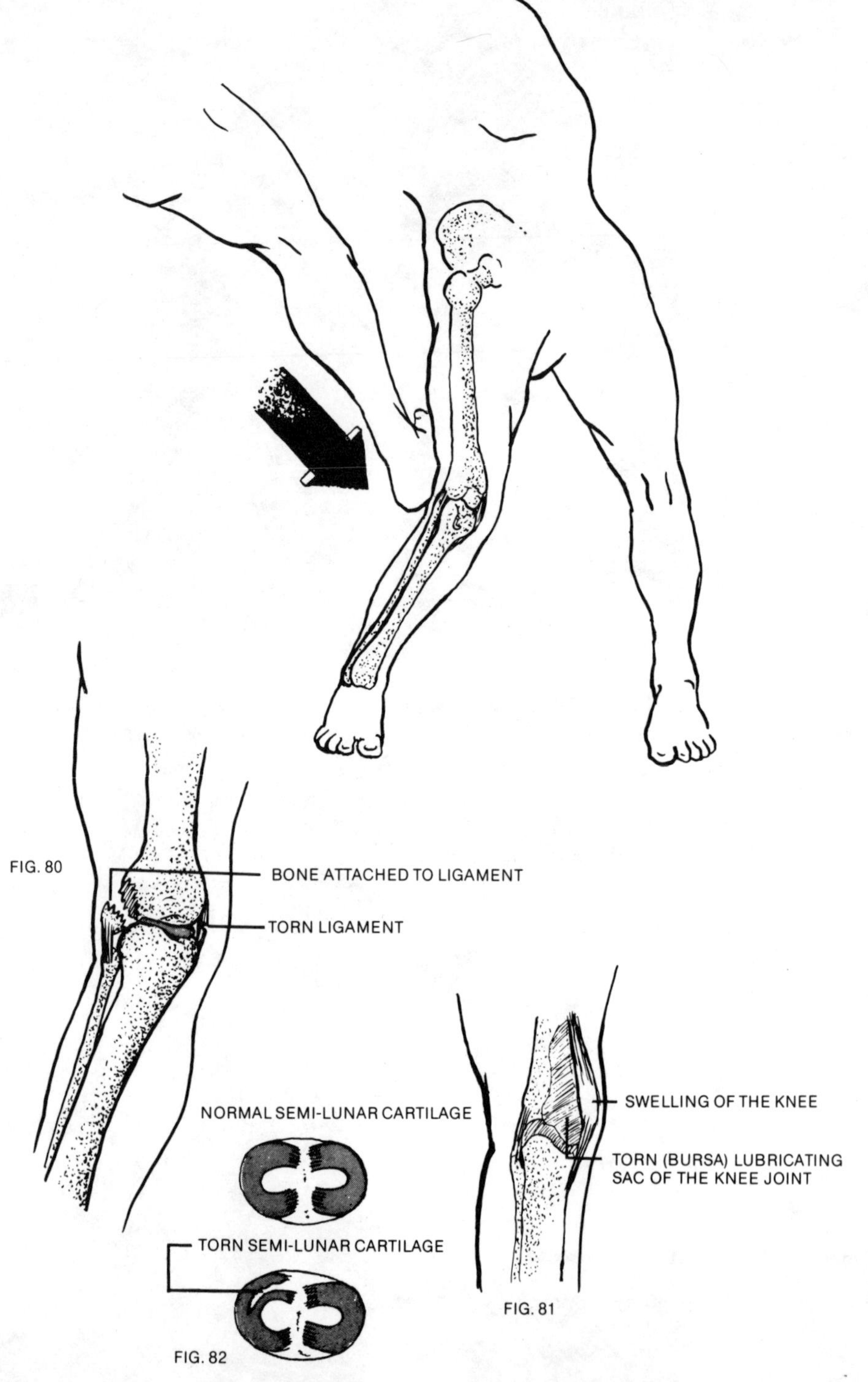

FIG. 80

FIG. 81

FIG. 82

WEAPON: Knife thrust (side of the foot)
TARGET: The side of the knee joint

Medical Implications

I. A LIGHT TO HEAVY SPRAIN will cause a tender or strained sensation in the knee joint, which is a result of the muscles and ligaments being stretched to their maximum elasticity. There will be painful movement and stiffness of the knee joint for quite some time.

II. SURFACE LACERATIONS (ABRASIONS) of the skin will occur if you are wearing hard soled shoes when you are attacked.

III. RUPTURED BLOOD VESSELS should be a result regardless of the strength of the kick. The larger vessels would be broken if it were a very forceful blow. There would be a large balloon or walnut like deformity (hematoma) pushing out wherever the blood vessel was torn.

IV. A TORN BURSA (lubricating sac that covers the lining of the knee joint) will occur very easily if it were pinched or abraded against any portion of the nearby bone surface, thus spilling the lubricating fluid under the skin and creating the usual grotesque, lumpy, or swollen appearance extending from the front to the back of the knee.

V. ABRADED AND TORN SEMI-LUNAR CARTILAGE is one of the most painful results that would follow (especially if the attacker had most of his weight on the forward foot and the knee was relatively straight at the moment of impact). This will come about by one bone grinding across the other in a sharp digging manner. The semi-lunar cartilage is the cushion of the knee joint. It aids in the smooth movement that exists when you walk or stoop down to pick up something from the floor. If the injury were bad enough, it could require surgical removal and/or repositioning of the cartilage fragments.

VI. AN AVULSION FRACTURE WITH TORN LIGAMENTS represents probably the most pictorial result that we can illustrate easily. If you will imagine a wire cable being plastered to a wall and then ripped loose after it was dried, consequently pulling a large chunk of attached plaster with it, then you can guess the painful results when a ligament has been ripped loose, pulling with it the bony insertion that normally adheres to the thigh bone (femur). This is possible when your foot hits above the joint and continues to scrape down the outside surface of the knee joint until it strikes the natural depression made by the two connecting bones (tibia and femur) and rips the ligament from its fixed position.

23

Striking the Shin Bone

Against a right hand knife thrust, defender sidesteps to the inside and simultaneously parries the arm away and cocks left leg for a kick.

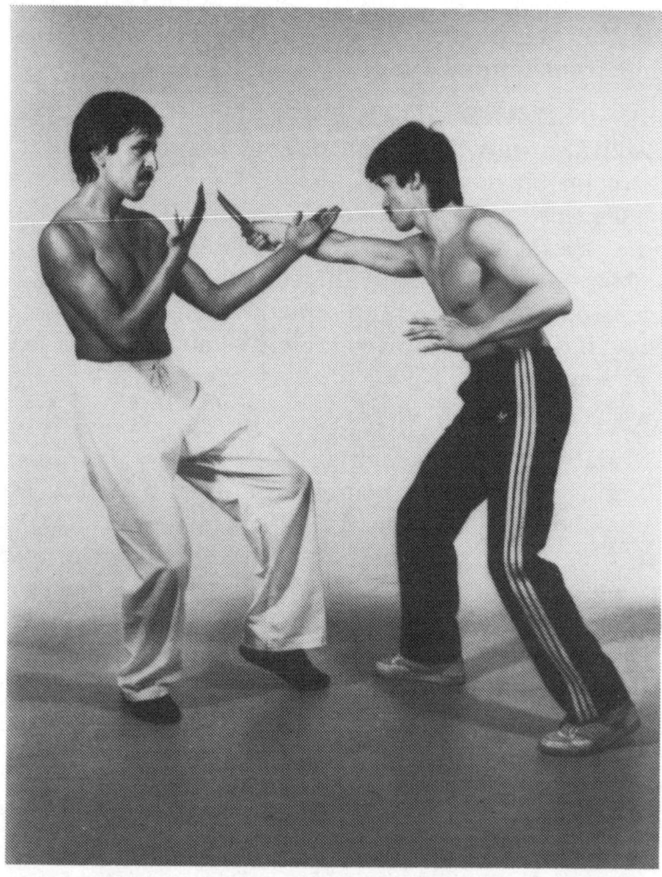

Defender maintains a check against the armed hand and strikes with side of his foot to the attacker's shin while pivoting away from the knife. This technique was completed in 4/10 of one second.

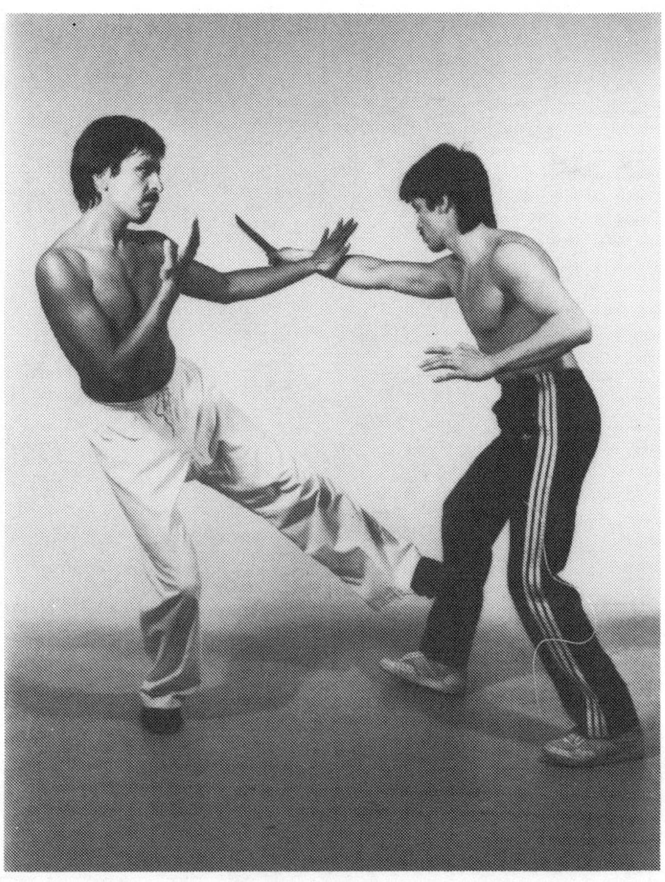

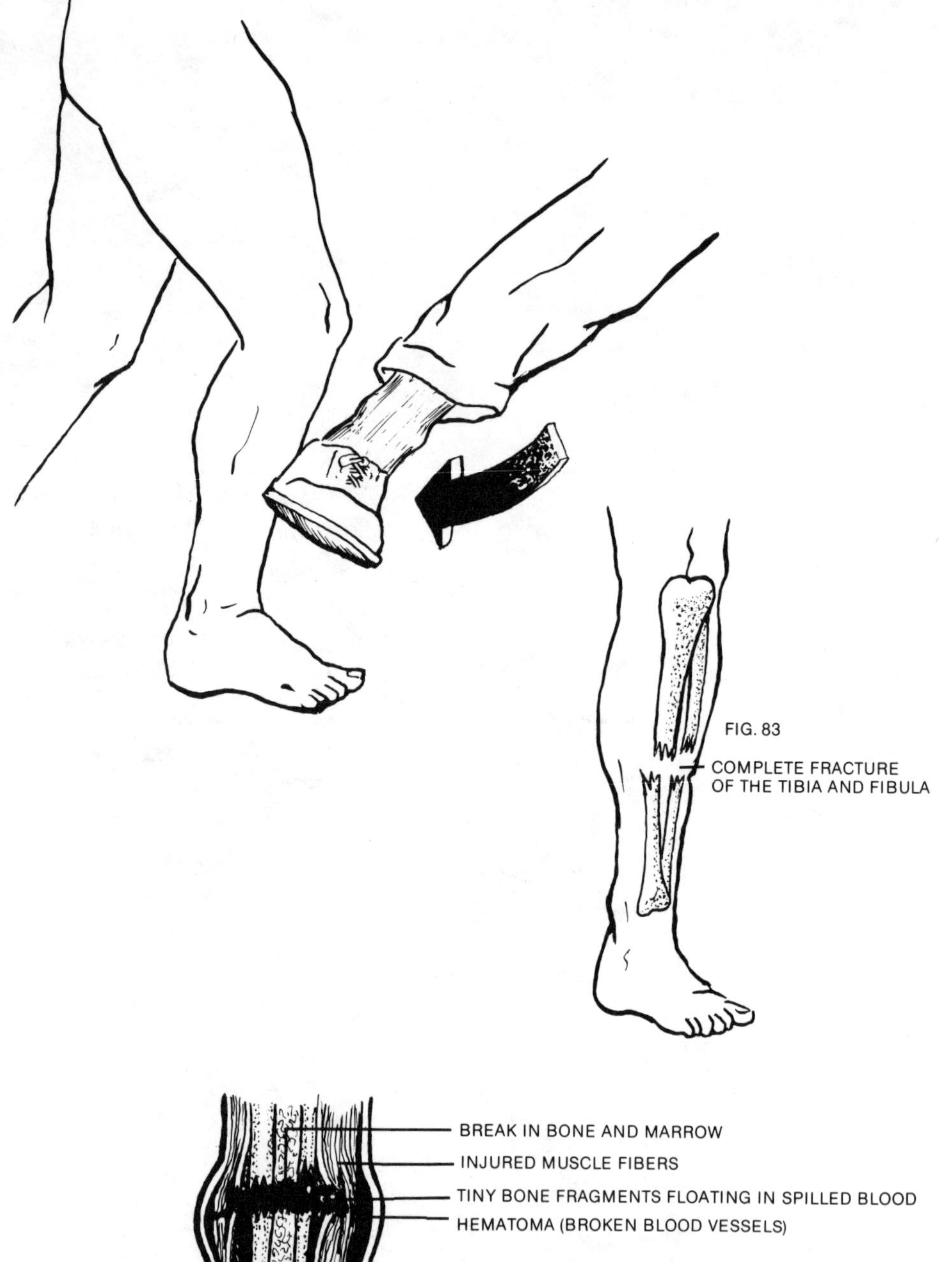

BLOW UP OF FRACTURED BONE
FIG. 84

WEAPON: Side of foot
TARGET: Shin bone

Medical Implications

I. Without a shoe, it is doubtful a complete break in the tibia or fibula will occur. But, if the kick is done with a hard soled shoe, it will easily fracture one or both bones of the lower limb, depending on the angle and solidity of the opponent's limb just prior to contact of the kick. The fracture is sometimes compounded soon after injury by the person's effort to stand and walk. If only one bone is fractured, the other bone will act as a splint, and, if the fracture is not a severe one, slight pressure can be applied (with great pain) for balance with most of the weight on the uninjured leg. Nauseating pain and inability to exert the slightest degree of pressure on the limb are companions of a complete fracture of the tibia and fibula.

II. A large area of blood spilled from the many torn blood vessels (hematoma) will form around the fracture site and create a huge swelling of the lower limb (Figure 84).

III. "Arterial embolism" is any abnormal particle carried in the vessel which becomes lodged in a vessel too small to permit its passage. The particles may be identified as a blood clot from another part of the body, fat, bacteria, bile or missils (bone) which cause circulatory failure of a section of the body, gangrene, or ultimately death.

In the case of a severe fracture of the shin where there are many tiny bone splinters, and many disrupted particles of fat (that normally lie between the layers of skin) there is a good possibility of these tiny particles finding their way into a torn blood vessel and lodging in a narrow part of the vessel. This is a threat whenever a bone has shattered into many fragments.

24

Striking the Achilles Tendon

Against a right cross, defender steps to the outside, grabs the attacker's right arm and cocks his leg to strike the attacker's right knee.

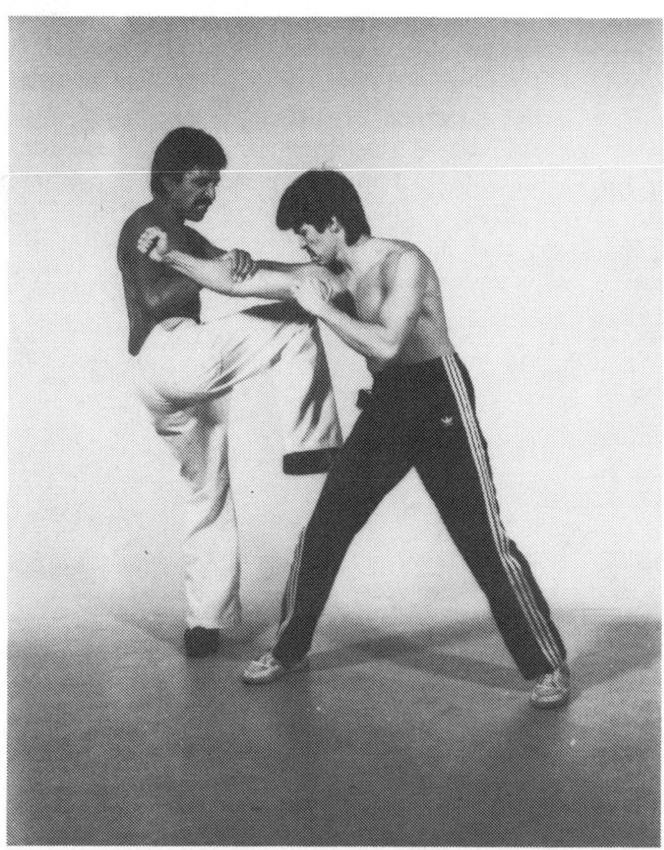

Holding on to the arm, defender drives the attacker's knee to the ground with the side of his foot.

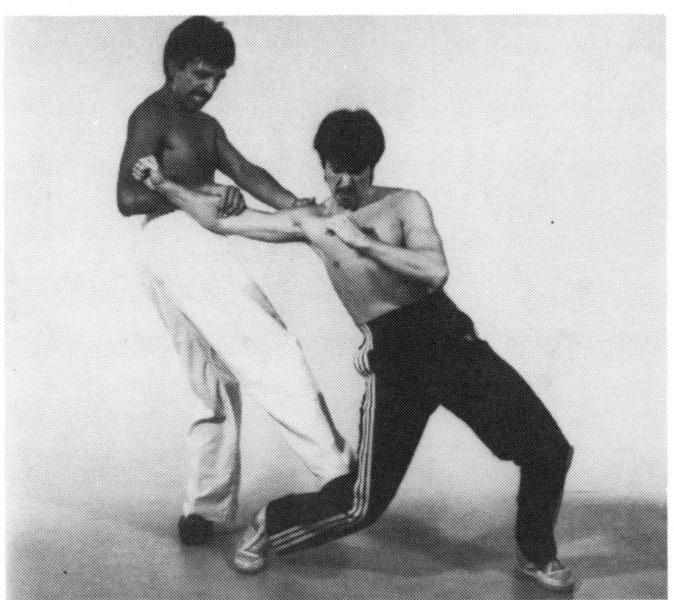

Defender pivots and stomps with his right heel onto attacker's achillies tendon. This technique was completed in 8/10 of one second.

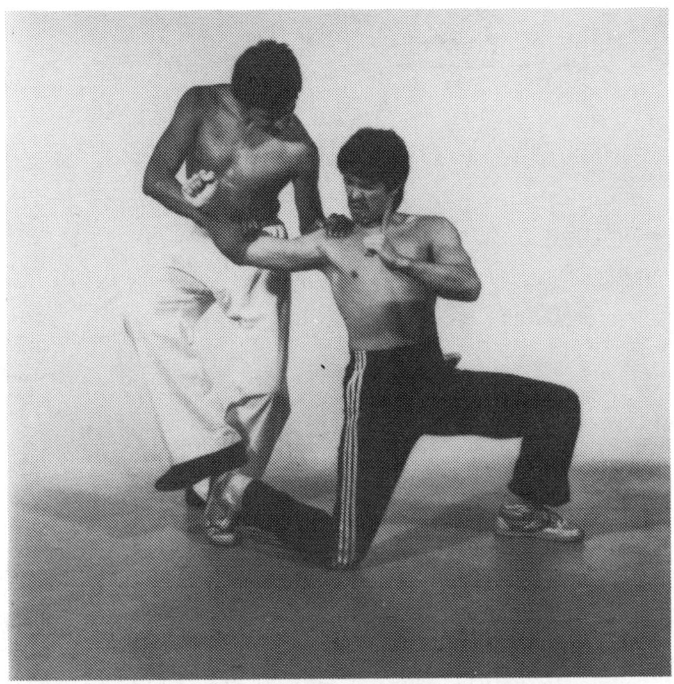

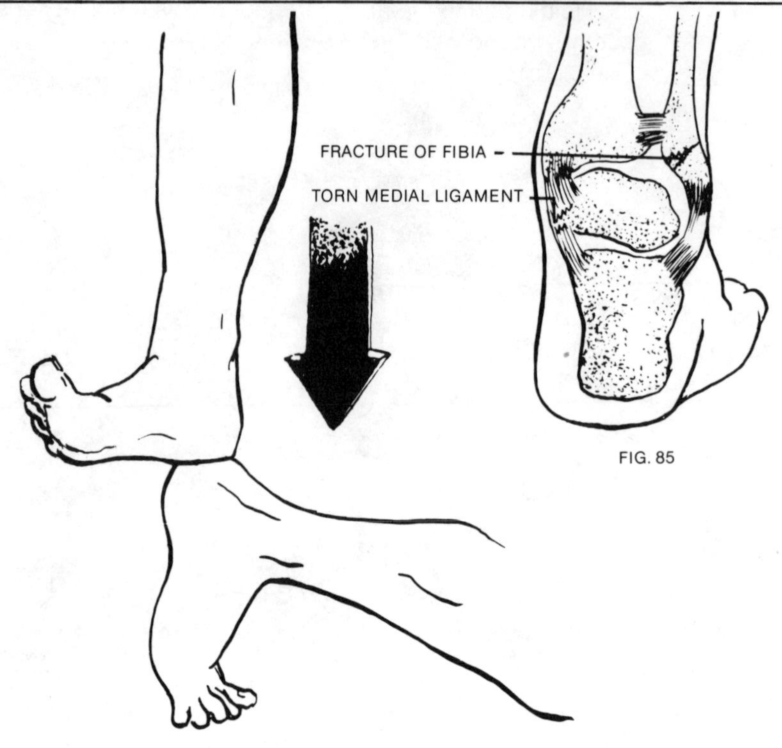

FIG. 85

FIG. 86

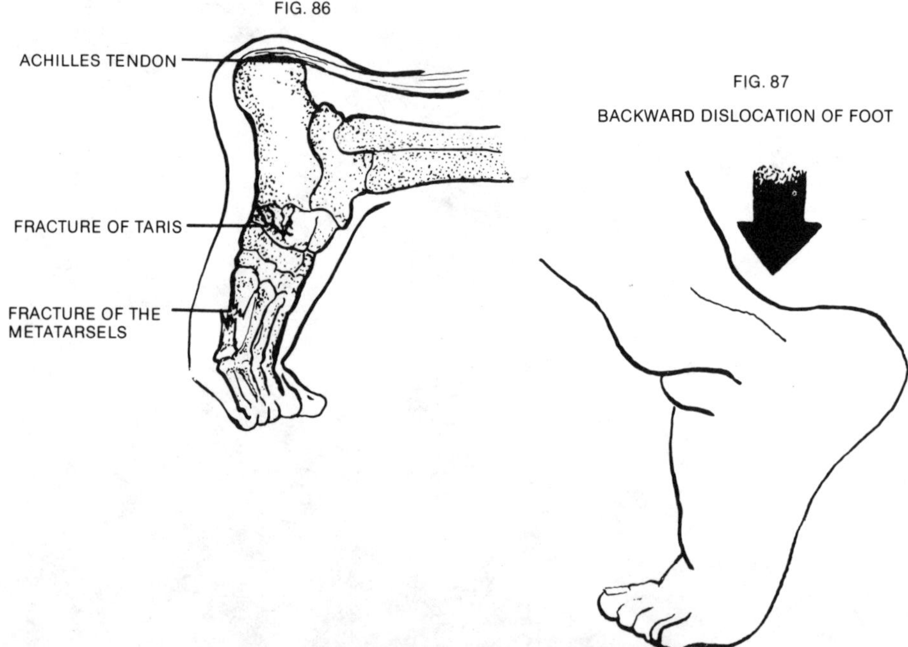

FIG. 87

BACKWARD DISLOCATION OF FOOT

WEAPON: Bottom of Foot
TARGET: Achilles tendon

Medical Implications

I. A sprained ankle is the least traumatic injury caused by a stomp with the foot in this position. Sprains are partially or completely torn ligaments, tendons and muscles. Sometimes they are just stretched to their limit and cause a great deal of ache and sharp pains when light pressure is applied.

II. Any combination of fractures of the tibia, fibula, tarsus and metatarsals (bones of the foot and ankle) will be present when the blow is struck with full force. An extreme swelling (hematoma) from many lacerated veins will grow so big as to make setting of the broken bones very difficult to manipulate into their original positions. Walking on the injured foot will be an impossiblity. Shock, nausea, and vomiting with possible loss of consciousness are immediate possibilities.

III. Backward dislocation of the foot (Fig. 87) is possible when the blow strikes the upper portion of the ankle. The tibia and fibula are thrust down toward the ground, virtually leaving the rest of the foot in its vertical position. The achilles tendon and many other ligaments and muscles will be ripped away from their fixed positions.

25
Shock

The term SHOCK will be present in a great many of the sections. Defining shock is not a simple task because much is known about it, but much is yet undiscovered. I will touch on only four closely related types of shock: (1) wound shock (2) hemorrhagic shock (3) septic shock (4) psychogenic shock.

(1) WOUND SHOCK may include all open type of wounds which result in CIRCULATORY FAILURE due to severe injury.

(2) HEMORRHAGIC SHOCK is generally a massive internal hemorrhage (loss of blood and plasma) with minimal injury. This usually refers to a key blood vessel that does not seal itself but continues to leak blood and plasma under the skin or into the body cavity without any immediate symptons. Weakness, shortness of breath, cold and clammy skin, sweating, greyness of the skin (pallor), thirst (due to the salivary glands ceasing to perform in their normal function), coma and death can occur within twenty-four hours.

(3) SEPTIC SHOCK is circulatory failure due to a host of infections. This is a later complication of injury (days or weeks after the initial injury).

(4) PSYCHOGENIC SHOCK is the most complicated of all types to define because it is a product of environment (society) and unpleasant past experiences (traumatic experiences). Slowing of the heart with a decrease in blood pressure (circulatory failure) when hearing unpleasant tidings and seeing objects of horror or the flow of blood, etc., is a social or individual development and usually ends with unconsciousness.

In summary, shock stems from either direct or indirect circulatory failure. Direct circulatory failure pertaining to the physical self (physical wound) and indirect circulatory failure pertaining to the mental self (psychologic trauma).

Death to the individual results when enough vital cells have died. Thus, and individual may die of anoxia (inadequate supply of oxygen) or uremia (toxic presence of urinary constituents in the blood) many days after all signs of shock have disappeared; or he may die of irreparable brain damage despite normal treatment for shock.

26
Principals of First Aid and Pain Reduction

Principals of Temporary First Aid and Pain Reduction

We are concerned here only with the practical aspects of temporary first aid and pain reduction. This then is supplementary to the preceeding chapters. Because the symptoms and the trauma are so explicitly described, I will not dwell on them in this section. The term "temporary first aid" must first be defined: As only that which is necessary to aid the victim until professional help can be given. Mainly comforting the victim; making sure there is not any unnecessary compounding of the injury; transporting the victim if applicable—all within the limits of the law. In other words, we are not going to practice medicine without a license.

The law may be somewhat different in various parts of the United States, but generally it is compatible with the Good Samaritan Act enforced all over the world—and so we will limit our approach to temporary first aid accordingly.

Liability for Emergency Care

Some states have enacted laws referred to as "Good Samaritan Acts." These laws limit or exclude liability for persons providing emergency medical or first aid treatment to the injured. In some states, these acts only protect licensed medical practitioners and not laymen. Most states still, however, apply rules of general negligence to all persons providing any form of treatment to an injured party despite the circumstances, emergency or otherwise. What this means is that any person providing care or first aid will be responsible to the injured party for mistakes or mistreatment, causing injury or aggravating pre-existing injury due to a lack of "reasonable care" in providing the emergency treatment. In other words, if a person is not well versed or qualified to administer first aid, then his exposure to liability for negligence is great.

The question arises as to a person's duty to come to another's aid if they are suffering from a potentially fatal injury that could be averted by emergency first aid. Surprisingly, a duty exists to provide first aid in this situation only in a limited number of circumstances. The law creates a duty upon persons enjoying a "special relationship" with the injured party to come to his aid. Such a "special relationship" exists between family members, employees and employers, in some cases, and when the injuries sustained were caused by the acts of the potential rescuer.

Other special relationships are possible and usually hinge on some social or moral community standard requiring a "reasonably prudent" person to act, i.e. a coach/player relationship. Unfortunately, the circumstances that lead to the conclusion that a duty to affirmatively act and provide first aid are quite often analyzed after the fact in a court of law. Barring a special relationship, there is no affirmative duty for an innocent bystander to provide emergency first aid and he or she does so at their own risk.

The temporary first aid measures offered here are intended for the use of a professional martial art instructor during supervised practice and, of course, may be used by the layman as needed. The following is an outline for general procedures in treating for temporary first aid:

1. Observe the victim.
2. Ask simple questions of the victim or witnesses.
3. Have the victim sit or lie down if he is standing.
4. Do not allow a crowd to hover around victim.
5. Make victim comfortable.
6. If needed start to apply pain reducing measures.
7. Expect shock—take preventive action.
8. Ask permission to treat victim if needed.
9. Get help: family, professional or a nearby person.
10. Advise professional follow-up.

1. "Observe the victim" to determine if temporary first aid is required.
    - A. Look for breathing and pulse signs if victim is unconscious (apply CPR if needed).
    - B. Look for external bleeding or abrasions (apply pressure to arteries: Fig. #1).
        1. Remember the three types of external bleeding signs:
            - a. Artery (spurts) carries blood away from the heart.
            - b. Vein (slow) steady and dark red, carries blood to heart.
            - c. Capillary (oozes) connects veins or artery.
    - C. Look for bone or skin deformities (indications of broken bones or broken blood vessels).
    - D. Look for signs of shock or the precursor of psychological shock. Remember common signs of shock are cold and clammy skin, light palor, slow or dull response, dizziness, diminished hearing or ringing

Fig. 1 Basic pressure points for controlling arterial bleeding.

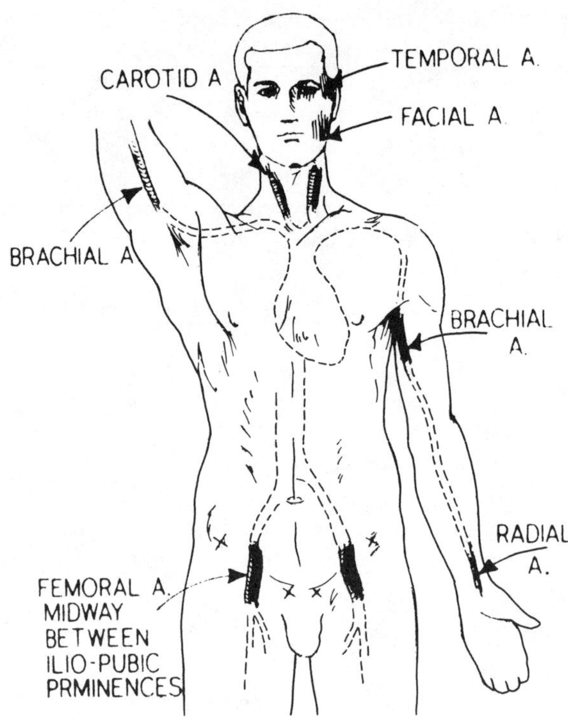

Fig. 2 Support victim at elbow and back of the neck when walking to sit or lie down to avoid further injury if victim faints. Elevate the feet in treatment for common shock.

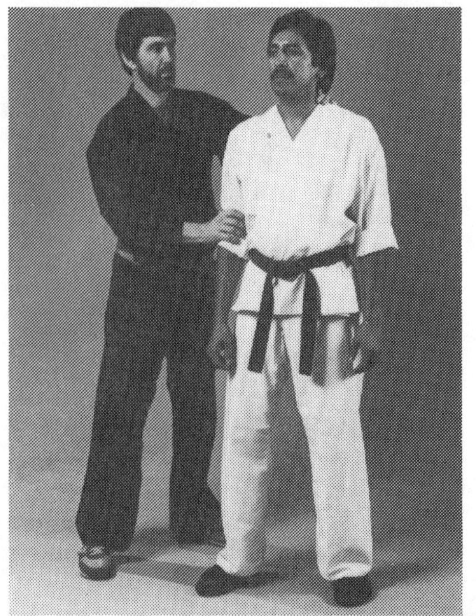

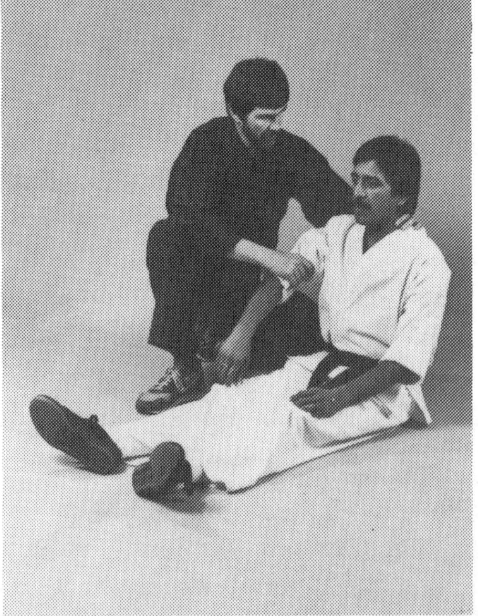

Fig. 3 When a head injury is suspected—elevate the head only—in treatment for common shock.

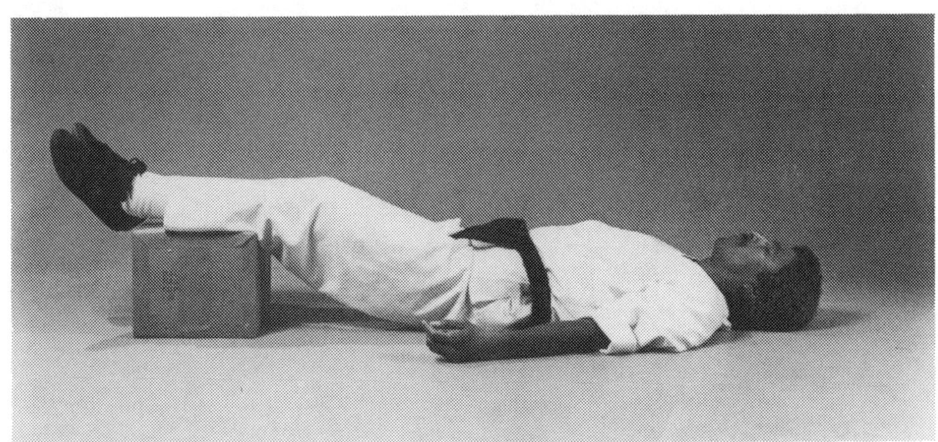

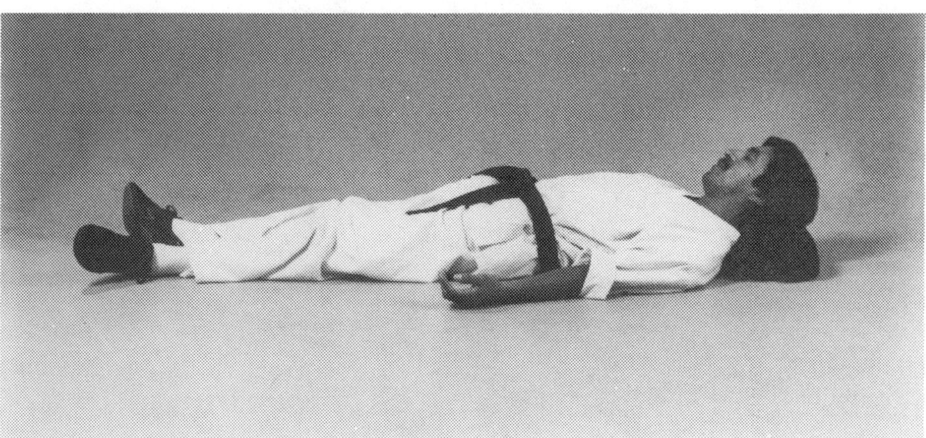

Fig. 4 The pupil on the left is dilated, as is sometimes seen in shock, stroke or brain injury. The pupil on the right is constricted as it reacts to light.

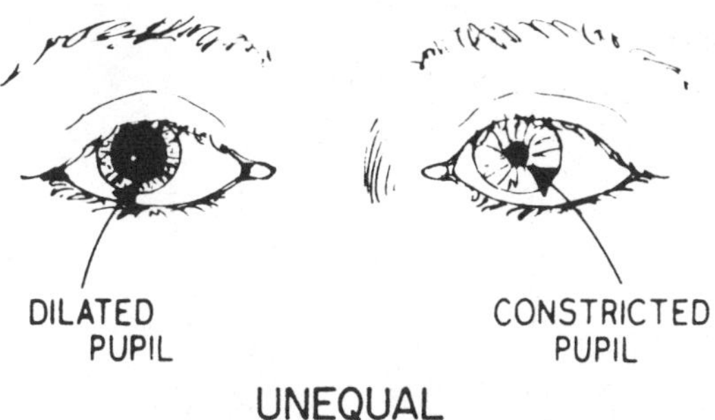

Fig. 5
A. Triangular bandage, used as a sling, is placed under the arm after the elbow is gently bent to a comfortable position. The pointed end of the sling is at the elbow and the two ends are placed behind the neck and tied.
B. The pointed end is pinned to the front of the sling.
C. The swathe (a separate piece of folded triangular gauze or material) is wrapped around the body to secure the injured arm.

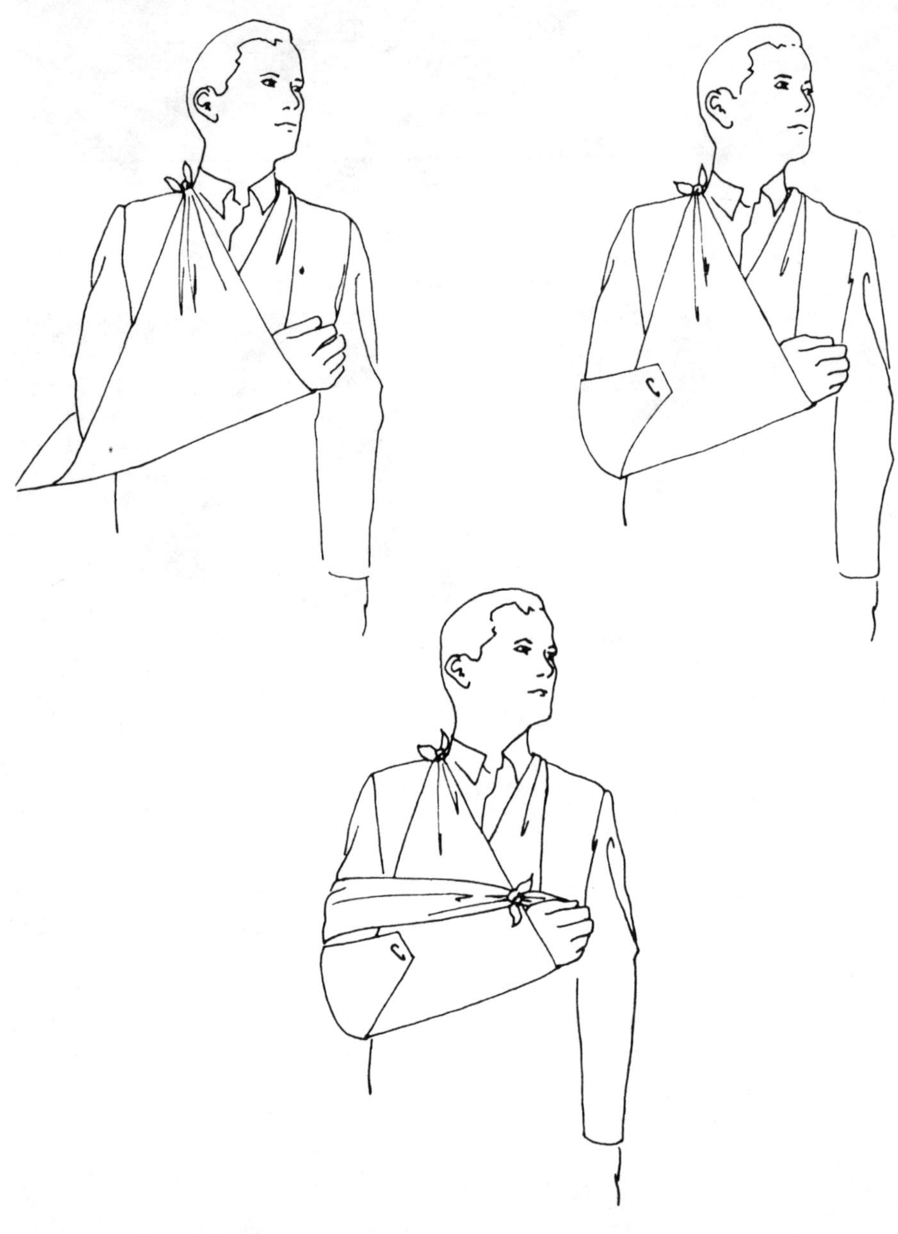

in the ears, feeling of physical weakness. Shock occurs in some degree with all injuries. In an excitable or nervous personality, psychological shock will certainly follow especially if the injury is a graphic one or if graphic comments are made by observers which will stimulate the reaction and expedite and exaggerate any shock response.

2. "Ask the victim (if he or she is conscious) or witnesses (if victim is unconscious) simple and direct questions."
   A. What happened? (Determine what degree of impact violence occurred.)
   B. How do you feel? (The answer will lead you to the next question.)

Then depending upon the type of injury, proceed with additional and more precise questioning.

Remember: The symptoms are descriptively inherent in each chapter and should be studied with a common sense approach. So if you understand the trauma and the symptoms, you will be able to ask the appropriate questions.

Example: Suspected spinal injury (neck—as in chapter 9). Lie the victim down flat on his back. Be sure to assist him to prevent further injury (See Fig. #2). Then proceed to ask questions using the common sense approach. Can you breath all right? (Is the vagas or phrenic nerve injured?); Do you have a tingling sensation or numbness anywhere? (pressure on a nerve or severed nerve); Can you move your toes, fingers, etc.? The answers to these questions will indicate how severe the damage and what appropriate action, if any, should follow.

Caution: In any severe injury (especially spinal injuries), let the professionals move and transport the victim.

3. "Have the victim lie or sit down if he is standing."
   This measure is to control and lessen any further trauma to the injury. Also, because shock does occur in varying degrees, in many instances the victim can faint for no apparent reason and compound the injury (See Fig. #2).
4. "Do not allow a crowd to hover around victim."
   Comments overheard by the victim could spark a shock reaction or panic.
5. "Make victim comfortable."
   Psychological comfort is of the utmost importance and can be influenced by your calmness and care. Maintaining physical contact as well as eye contact is reassuring to the victim. Physically position the victim according to the type of injury. For instance, if you suspect a severe head injury (as in chapter 3), support victim's head slightly with a pillow when lying down so that internal blood will not rush to the injury and compound it (See Fig. #3).
6. "If needed start to apply pain reducing measures."
   We will use a combination of eastern and western methods of pain reduction.
   A. A sprain or fractured limb should be elevated to reduce swelling and pain.

B. Ice or cold is the primary means to reduce pain and swelling. Cold should be applied off and on for the first 48 hours.

1. "Physiology of wound healing."
Marked swelling delays the process of healing, it restricts circulation, retards local metabolism and favors bacterial growth. Mild localized swelling, however, is considered to be beneficial especially *48 hours* later as in most hematomas. The application of ice during the first few hours following the injury and continuing up to 48 hours (as needed) and then after 48 hours the application of heat is the recommended procedure in hematomas, myatomas, etc.

C. Pads, wraps, slings and splints aid in further reducing injury to the limb and act as a support system in place of the bone (Fig. #4).

D. Deep breathing will help create a feeling of well being and calm. Use sets of four to eight complete inhalations and exhalations.

E. Pressure points for relieving pain are used primarily in the Orient and effective in 96 percent of pain victims.

7. "Expect shock; take preventive action."
The basic treatment for shock is to lie a person down on his back and elevate the feet in order to increase bloodflow to the brain (See Fig. #3). The exception would be if the victim had a suspected head injury. In shock the blood flow to the skin is redirected inward toward the thoraic cavity—this is why the skin takes on a colorless hue and becomes cooler. The victim may also feel weak or faint. The body's natural survival system will draw blood away from the head and limbs in order to slow or stop the loss of blood from a wound. Remember to treat for psychological shock as in #1-D.

8. "Ask permission to treat the victim if needed."
If the person is conscious, ask permission to apply temporary first aid. Remember: This is to minimize the legal limitations set by the law and to notify the victim of your professional limitations. If the person is unconscious, you have the same potential legal limitations so you must use your own discretion on what limits to set for the situation.

9. "Advise Professional Follow-up."
You probably do not have the professional medical background to be responsible for a final diagnosis. It is better to be safe than sorry. Recovery and therapy should be evaluated by their own personal physician.

Simple First Aid Kit and Common Environmental Aids

1. Ice Bag
2. Assorted sizes of splints for arms, legs and fingers.
3. Arm slings for shoulder, elbow, forearm and wrist injuries.
4. Isopropyl alcohol for use as an antiseptic.
5. Plastic adhesive strips.
6. Elastic bandages for wrist, ankle and knee injuries.
7. Package of cotton balls (for cleaning cuts & abrasions).
8. Adhesive tape (for splints & sprains, etc.).
9. Gauze bandages (sterile).
10. Eye cup (an ordinary paper cup) to prevent subconscious touching of the injury.
11. Scissors (blunt ends) for cutting clothing away from the injury and for cutting materials needed.
12. Blanket (in treatment for shock). Folded for elevating head or feet.

Bibliography

CHAPTER 1.
a. *A Compilation of Paintings on Normal and Pathological Nervous Systems, With a Supplement on the Hypothalmus,* Vol. I. Frank H. Netter, Summit, N.J. CIBA Pharmaceutical Products Inc. 2nd Edition, Section 5.
b. *Callander's Surgical Anatomy* by Barry J. Anson and Walter G. Maddock. Philadelphia, W.B. Saunders. Chapter 1, 4th Edition.
c. *Cunningham's Textbook of Anatomy,* Tenth Edition, London Oxford University Press, New York, Toronto. (Facial Nerve).
d. *Atlas of Human Anatomy: Simplified,* by Gaynor Evans. Littlefield, Adams and Co., Patterson, N.J. Chapter 3.

CHAPTER 2.
a. *Callander's Surgical Anatomy,* Chapters 2 and 3, 3rd Edition, Chapter 2, 4th Edition.
b. *Atlas of Human Anatomy: Simplified,* Chapter 7.

CHAPTER 3.
a. *Callander's Surgical Anatomy,* Chapters 1 and 2, 4th Edition.
b. *A Compilation of Paintings on Normal and Pathological Nervous Systems, With a Supplement on the Hypothalmus,* Vol. I, 2nd Edition, Section 2.
c. *An Atlas of Head and Neck Surgery,* John M. Lore, Jr., MD. Saunders Co. Philadelphia & London. Section 5.
d. *Cunningham's Textbook of Anatomy,* 10th Edition. London, New York, Toronto, Oxford University Press. "The Skull," "The Blood, Vascular and Lymphatic Systems," "Arteries of the Head and Neck."

CHAPTER 4.
a. *Callander's Surgical Anatomy* by Barry J. Anson and Walter G. Maddock. Philadelphia, W.B. Saunders. 4th Edition, Chapter 1.

CHAPTER 5.
a. *Cunningham's Textbook of Anatomy,* Tenth Edition, pages 693-695.
b. *Fundamentals of Otolaryngology* by Lawrence R. Boies, MD. 3rd Edition, Saunders Co. Pages 289-290.
c. *An Atlas of Head and Neck Surgery,* Section 4.

CHAPTER 6.
a. *Fundamentals of Otolaryngology* 3rd Edition, Page 288.
b. *Callander's Surgical Anatomy,* 3rd Edition, Chapter 1.

CHAPTER 7.
a. *Fundamentals of Otolaryngology,* 3rd Edition, Pages 287-288.
b. *An Atlas of Head and Neck Surgery,* Section 5.
c. *Callander's Surgical Anatomy,* 4th Edition, Chapter 3.
d. *Christopher's Textbook of Surgery,* W.B. Saunders Co. Philadelphia & London. 7th Edition. Page 278.
e. *Cunningham's Textbook of Anatomy,* 10th Edition, Chapter 11.

CHAPTER 8.
a. *Management of Fractures and Disclocation: an Atlas* by Anthony S. De Plama. Philadelphia, W.B. Saunders Co. Vol. I, Part #1.
b. *Fundamentals of Otolaryngology* Pages 323, 389, 393.
c. *Callander's Surgical Anatomy,* 4th Edition, Chapters 7, 8 and 9.
d. *Cunningham's Textbook of Anatomy,* 10th Edition. "The Peripheral Nervous System," "The Digestive System."
e. *Christopher's Textbook of Surgery,* 8th Edition, Chapter #10.

CHAPTER 9.
a. *A Compilation of Paintings on Normal and Pathological Nervous Systems, With a Supplement on the Hypothalmus,* 2nd Edition, Section #5.
b. *Management of Fractures and Dislocation: an Atlas,* Vol. I, Part1.
c. *Callander's Surgical Anatomy,* 4th Edition, Chapters 8 and 26.

CHAPTER 10.
a. *Callander's Surgical Anatomy,* 4th Edition, Chapters 8 and 27.
b. *Management of Fractures and Dislocations: an Atlas,* Vol. I, Part 1.
c. *Cunningham's Textbook of Anatomy,* 10th Edition, "The Peripheral Nervous System."

CHAPTER 11.
a. *Cunningham's Textbook of Anatomy,* 10th Edition.
b. *Christopher's Textbook of Surgery,* 8th Edition, Chapters 4, 15, 17, 18 and 19.
c. *Callander's Surgical Anatomy,* 8th Edition, Chapter 15.

CHAPTER 12.
a. *Management of Fractures and Dislocations: an Atlas,* Vol. 1, Parts 1 and 2.
b. *Callander's Surgical Anatomy,* 4th Edition, Chapter 12.
c. *Cunningham's Textbook of Anatomy,* 10th Edition, "The Respiratory System."

CHAPTER 13.
a. *Callander's Surgical Anatomy,* 4th Edition, Chapter 15.
b. *Cunningham's Textbook of Anatomy,* 10th Edition, "Myology."

CHAPTER 14.
a. *Archives of Surgery,* Vol. 92, No. 3, March 1966, Page 362. "Delayed Rupture of the Spleen."
b. *Christopher's Textbook of Surgery,* Chapter 21.
c. *Cunningham's Textbook of Anatomy,* 10th Edition, "The Blood, Vascular and Lymphatic Systems."

CHAPTER 15.
a. *Cunningham's Textbook of Anatomy,* 10th Edition, "The Urogenital System."
b. *Callander's Surgical Anatomy,* 4th Edition, Chapters 14 and 15.
c. *Christopher's Textbook of Surgery,* 8th Edition, Chapter 22.

CHAPTER 16.
a. *Management of Fractures and Disclocations: an Atlas,* Vol. I, Parts 1 and 2.

CHAPTER 17.
a. *Management of Fractures and Dislocations: an Atlas,* Vol. I, Part 1.
b. *Callander's Surgical Anatomy,* 4th Edition, Chapters 16 and 17.
c. *Christopher's Textbook of Surgery,* 8th Edition, Chapters 16 and 22.
d. *Atlas of Human Anatomy: Simplified,* Chapter 8.

CHAPTER 18.
a. *Callander's Surgical Anatomy,* 4th Edition, Chapters 16 and 18.
b. *Christopher's Textbook of Surgery,* 8th Edition, Chapter 23.

CHAPTER 19.
a. *A Compilation of Paintings on Normal and Pathological Nervous Systems With a Supplement on the Hypothalmus,* Vol. I, Section 5.
b. *Management of Fractures and Dislocations: an Atlas,* Vol. I, Part 1.
c. *Callander's Surgical Anatomy,* 4th Edition, Chapters 36 and 37.

CHAPTER 20.
a. *Management of Fractures and Dislocations: an Atlas,* Vol. II, Part 2.
b. *Callander's Surgical Anatomy,* 4th Edition, Chapters 36 and 37.

CHAPTER 21.
a. *Management of Fractures and Dislocations: an Atlas,* Vol. II, Part 2.
b. *Callander's Surgical Anatomy,* 4th Edition, Part 35.
c. *Management of Fractures and Dislocations: an Atlas,* Vol. I, Part 1.
d. *Christopher's Textbook of Surgery,* 8th Edition, Chapter 35.

CHAPTER 22.
a. *Management of Fractures and Dislocations: an Atlas,* Vol. II, Part 2.
b. *Callander's Surgical Anatomy,* 4th Edition, Chapter 35.
c. *Christopher's Textbook of Surgery,* 8th Edition, Chapter 25.

CHAPTER 23.
a. *Management of Fractures and Dislocations: an Atlas,* Vol. II, Part 2, Vol. I, Part 2.
b. *Callander's Surgical Anatomy,* 3rd Edition, Chapter 31.
c. *Christopher's Textbook of Surgery,* 8th Edition, "Arterial Embolism."

CHAPTER 24.
a. *Callander's Surgical Anatomy,* 4th Edition, Chapter 39.
b. *Management of Fractures and Dislocations: an Atlas,* Vol. II, Part 2 and Vol. I, Part 1.

CHAPTER 25.
Emergency Care and Transportation of the Sick and Injured, by The Committee on Injuries, American Academy of Orthopaedic Surgeons.

UNIQUE LITERARY BOOKS OF THE WORLD